# Praise for *Living Agelessly*

"… a how-to guide for surviving life's pitfalls as we Baby Boomers venture into the vast and uncharted waters of senior citizenship… Living Agelessly" has helped reinforce my doctors' prescriptions for better diet, more exercise and how important a positive outlook can be. Altoonian explores the spiritual connection between good nutrition, exercise and a positive, forward-looking attitude. It's really the ABC's of fearlessly, even eagerly, moving into another phase of our lives filled with time to do the things we never could fit into our work-crammed lives before, including travel, volunteering and grandchildren. It's a book anyone already at or approaching retirement should keep handy on their bookshelves and it's a tremendous resource for those who have aging parents.
— JIM REEVES, FORT WORTH STAR-TELEGRAM

"… a fount of information written clearly, succinctly, and with style. I couldn't put it down. Not only is it an interesting read, the book is also an important tool for every age… *Living Agelessly* shows us how to grow older with increased awareness, greater power, and far more success. This is truly a book I will refer to constantly." — BARBARA POPE MUSSER, LMFT, LICENSED MARRIAGE AND FAMILY THERAPIST

"… a must-have for anyone with aging parents, or who is approaching retirement age themselves or is already retired. Well-organized sections on health & fitness, preparing for retirement, and safety issues make it easy to find information. Some of the chapters I found particularly helpful (I'm nearing retirement age) were the ones on travel and volunteering… numerous ideas on how to interact with your grandkids in today's world …

"One of my favorite features about *Living Agelessly* is its emphasis on mind-body connections. It stresses the importance of a healthy body and positive attitude… the resources section at the end of the book provides hundreds of websites and phone numbers of organizations dedicated to working with retirees…" — LIBRARY THING EARLY REVIEWER

"… the most engaging overview of *aging gracefully* you'll find… (this) practical guide is based, not only on personal experience, but five years feedback from sometimes desperate but always enthusiastic readers of her column on aging. She knows what readers need to know, and provides practical, easy-to-understand answers. She's also fun to read, even on topics that are extremely serious." — LAEL MORGAN, UNIVERSITY OF TEXAS AT ARLINGTON

"… contains hundreds and hundreds of helpful and economical insights distilled from Ms Altoonian's award winning, 'Dear Ageless' column… pages of links to helpful websites and other resources for anyone approaching retirement, just retired, or needing to deal with the last mile. The emphasis is on maximizing life, not squeezing life as we move into a fixed income lifestyle. — LIBRARY THING EARLY REVIEWER

"… the best—the one and only guide I would ever need to gracious, graceful aging… Kudos to Linda Altoonian! She has given each of us a compass to age well and live fully." — CAROLYN LESSER, AUTHOR, CONSULTANT, SPEAKER

"… easy to read and understand and will be a great asset to those who will be caring for aging family and friends… clear and concise with many resources… a great blueprint for those of us who are "baby boomers" to make preparations in advance of needing things." — JANE ODERBERG, LMSW, CANCER CARE SERVICES

"… simple, easy to understand, and extremely practical. Linda Altoonian has given the reader a wealth of information without creating a tome that one must wade through in order to dig out the information. She has done the hard work of sorting out all these tough issues, and anyone who reads *Living Agelessly* will immediately see how valuable this work is. After all, all of us age, so why not learn how to do it gracefully…" — DR. JAMES M. REEVES, PASTOR

# Living
# Agelessly

*Answers to Your Most Common Questions*
*About Aging Gracefully*

Linda Altoonian

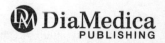 DiaMedica
PUBLISHING

DiaMedica Publishing, 150 East 61st Street, New York, NY 10065
Visit our website at *www.diamedicapub.com*

Library of Congress Cataloging-in-Publication Data available from the Publisher.

ISBN: 978-0-9793564-4-5

Note to Readers
This book is not a substitute for medical advice and assistance. The judgment of individual physicians and other medical specialists who know you and who manage the treatment of any medical issues you may have is essential.

Editor: Jessica Bryan
Designed and typeset by: TypeWriting

# Dedication and Acknowledgments

To my parents for giving me the reason to begin this phase of my life.

To my family for their encouragement.

To my life group for its continual support.

To Brad Porter for his technical help.

To my publisher, Dr. Diana M. Schneider, for her help throughout this process.

To my dearest friend, Barb Musser, whose life-long loyalty has been a true gift.

# About the Author

Linda Altoonian is an award-winning writer, whose Dear Ageless column has appeared regularly in the *Fort Worth Star-Telegram*, *Winslow Mail*, *Golden Gazette*, and on the AP Wire Service. She has been the editor-in-chief of various national magazines, including the *Mickey Mantle* and *Selena* Collector's Editions, and has been a consultant to advertising agencies and publishers.

Today, Linda writes and also teaches journalism. Her excellence in the classroom was recognized by the Press Women of Texas, who voted her State Journalism Teacher of the Year.

She is the recipient of many other prestigious awards, including the *Time Magazine* Award for Most Outstanding Publication in the Nation, the President's Service Award for her work in magazines, and an Editor's Choice Award for her writing.

She has had numerous articles and stories published in anthologies. This is her first full-length book.

With time out for extensive travel, Linda has resided in Texas for almost 25 years, where she raised two great kids and cared for her parents, who served as the inspiration for this book.

# Contents

# Preface

Baby boomers, and their parents, are the fastest growing segments of the population. We are 81 million strong, and have shaped every aspect of American life for decades. We have been the moving force in changing or creating new industries (designer clothes and bottled water). We have exploded existing markets (flavored coffee and computers), and have destroyed others (typewriters and cloth diapers).

Also called the "sandwich generation," many baby boomers are raising children at the same time that they are caring for their aging parents, who will live 10 to 15 years on average longer than the generations before them. Baby boomers are racing from day care centers for their kids to nursing centers for their parents—and sometimes their grandparents.

Every year, 4 million baby boomers turn 50, but we refuse to be downsized or ignored. Controlling over 48 percent of all discretionary purchases, baby boomers are the most educated, proactive, and affluent consumer group in North America. We will read, do, and buy whatever it takes to remain as young and healthy as possible, for as long as possible.

Determined to age less and age well, we are taking better care of ourselves, so age 60 looks and feels more like 40. Because we are living longer, we are reinventing ourselves in the workplace, and are far more interested in keeping active than sitting in any rocking chair.

The "Me" generation is wealthier than our children are likely to be, and we are more likely to use our money to create a golden retirement rather than will it to others. Our attitude about aging is different from any previous generation—and attitude dictates how successfully a person will grow older.

*Living Agelessly* was written for anyone who wants to maximize health and create an independent and successful lifestyle. The suggestions in this book apply to young adults who are concerned about preparing better for the inevitable changes associated with growing older, to the sandwich generation that is juggling the care of children and aging parents, to baby boomers, and to those who are in their early years of retirement.

I have lived all of those stages but the last. For more than two decades, I happily attended to the lives of a very busy family, did volunteer work in the school and community, and was politically active. When my children were older, I began carving out a new career—writing for and editing magazines—the perfect work for remaining fully involved in my children's activities. When they began college, I added teaching journalism and advising publication staffs to my already full schedule. I had created an exciting career for myself, and it was my time to enjoy the new life I had fashioned.

The euphoria was short-lived. My parents were ill when they moved nearby, and the information I needed to solve their multiple problems was either lacking or too complicated. So, in order to be an informed advocate, I began researching various topics about aging. Then I decided to share my findings. This was the genesis of *Dear Ageless*—my newspaper column addressing the issues of growing older.

I soon found out that most of the letters to my advice column would not come from silver-haired readers. Instead, the letters come from younger people—the "baby boomers" who are either involved in caring for their aging parents or looking for ways to age more successfully themselves.

Surprisingly, I am also deluged with letters from the *children* of the baby boomers. They expect to live longer than earlier generations, and they do not want to be a burden to their children and grandchildren. They want to be healthy; they expect to be caregivers, and they want to have enough money to pay their bills and enjoy what will be a long life after they stop working.

All of these age groups desire a source of expert information and top-notch referrals to enable them to fulfill their needs and accomplish their goals. Many readers have also asked that the column information be gathered into a single book that could serve as a comprehensive resource. *Living Agelessly* is the result of those requests. It addresses the questions that readers often ask: How can I stay healthy? How can I live with greater control and power in my life? How can I protect myself? How can I enjoy life more?

The most frequently asked questions sent to my column form the basis of the topics I chose for this book. They emphasize three broad areas:

▶ The desire for the latest information about optimizing nutrition, exercise, and other areas related to the best health possible, both in the present and in preparation for the future;

▶ The need to create a secure and enjoyable retirement—rich with wonderful relationships, interesting travel, and rewarding experiences; and

▶ Concern about the practical issues of growing older, both to prepare for your own greater comfort and for that of aging parents.

Reflecting this, the initial chapters deal with the broad topic of overall mental and physical health and wellness. The following chapters include such enjoyable topics as traveling (adults-only and with family), the special rewards of volunteering, and the unique role of grandparenting. These chapters will be of special interest to parents whose children are grown, and who are making the transition to retirement. The final chapters deal with the needs of older individuals, and cover such topics as home safety, driving issues, and caregiving.

I took care of my parents for almost five years before they passed away within six months of each other. I am still reeling from my emotions surrounding their care and passing, but I am also grateful. Had I not taken care of my own parents, I wouldn't have been so sympathetic to the problems of aging, and I wouldn't have created the column *Dear Ageless.*

In going through this process, I learned how to approach aging with more far more understanding and better preparation than my parents did, and I find great satisfaction in passing on this understanding, guidance, and information to my readers—my fellow baby boomers, their children, and their parents.

*Linda Altoonian*

# Introduction

*Living Agelessly* is divided into three sections. The initial chapters are directed to all age groups and address how to improve quality of life, how to stay healthy—mentally and physically—and how to slow the aging process and even reverse some of its effects.

The second section is directed both to readers who want to prepare for their future retirement and to those who want to enrich the retirement they already have.

The third section deals with a variety of issues that will help those in the sandwich generation—who might be juggling the care of their immediate families with the care of members of their extended family—the caregivers who have to care for themselves and for aged family members, and the seniors who are faced with the many challenges of growing older.

The book contains numerous tips and recommendations, both within the text and in the comprehensive Resources section, including useful books, telephone numbers of agencies and organizations, and websites that can be used for additional research. You will have at your fingertips resources that are current, cutting-edge, and incredibly supportive.

The letters I've included from my newspaper column are sometimes funny, sometimes poignant, but always at the heart of the matter. We are *all* growing older, and it's a tough process. Smart people enlist help to do it well. *Living Agelessly* is intended to provide that help.

The first chapter discusses the critical connection between the mind, body, and spirit. To achieve optimal health and happiness, to gain control of environment and relationships, and to exercise restraint over our emotions and reactions, we must not only understand the link between these parts of ourselves, but also we must unleash and integrate their power. What we think, say aloud, and choose to do determines who we are. If we are not satisfied with who we are or how things are going, then we need to make changes. This chapter will aid us in doing so.

Chapters 2 and 3 include the latest information about good nutrition—both macro- and micronutrients that can dramatically change how we look and feel. Here is the latest information about the power foods that create greater energy, stamina, and clarity; improve well-being and physical appearance; and battle disease and aging. This chapter demonstrates that even small changes in diet can make dramatic differences.

Chapter 4 addresses exercise, which is a challenge for even the healthiest among us. The excuses for not exercising are usually no time, no energy, or—in the case of the elderly—no strength. Very often, the truth is that we are not motivated. Unlike when we were children, when it was fun to exert our bodies, for most of us, exercise is just another chore to accomplish on our already too-full "To-Do List." This chapter discusses the latest theories about maximizing the benefit of exercise with a minimum commitment of time. It outlines simple ways to build in movement, increase strength and energy, and breathe our way to good health.

After learning how to look good and feel energized, the next section shows you how to shape a retirement that will be fun and fabulous, without having to be rich! In Chapter 5, you will learn how to visit an exotic location without paying a cent, how to tour Europe for a pittance, or how to cruise the world for a year for the same amount that you would spend for one year of assisted care—and you will have a lot more fun.

Lists of tips are available for traveling safely, traveling alone, or traveling for the first time. Travel does not have to be some far-off dream. You will learn how to make it a reality and have the time of your life.

If you started working when you were 16 and retired at 65, you will have worked for almost 50 years! That's a lot of time to live with a built-in structure, a goal-oriented direction, and measurable accomplishments and rewards. We work that long not just because we must, but also because it gives us a sense of importance and value, an opportunity to contribute our gifts to society, and a good reason for getting up in the morning.

After so many years of production, you are certainly entitled to a rest, and you might decide never to work again full time or even for money. However, if you stop making a contribution altogether after retirement, you might as well relegate yourself to a rocking chair and expect a quicker dccline. We all need to feel productive, valuable, and necessary to someone, or what reason would we have for wanting to go on?

The options for accomplishing these three goals—to be productive, valuable, and needed—are without limit. Chapter 6 shows you how to share with others the treasure of knowledge, expertise, and experience you have accumulated over a lifetime. They say "a mind is a terrible thing to waste." So is a well-lived life.

Chapter 7 addresses one of the most unique and special relationships possible. The relationship a grandparent has with a grandchild is perhaps the closest thing to a real miracle. You get to experience the pure love and adoration of a child without any of the responsibility. For the most part, you are free to conspire, have fun, and even "spoil" your grandchildren without any fear, and you can return them to your children when you're finally tuckered out from so much enjoyment. It truly is the best of all possible worlds!

There are considerations, however. You want to be sure that your home and property are safe for their visits. You will want to do activities with your grandchildren that make lifelong memories, and you will want to pass on the history and values of your family—the most important job of a grandparent. This chapter is full of ideas that will make their memory of you last for as long as *they* live.

Chapters 8 and 9 will enable you to make your home a safe environment for your family members and for yourself. As we grow older, our memory is not quite what it once was, and neither is our reaction time. It is critical to anticipate problems and solve them before someone is hurt. Included are many valuable suggestions, tip lists, and product recommendations for making your home the safe sanctuary it should be.

Giving up the car keys is perhaps one of the most difficult signposts of aging. It's the moment when people feel they are no longer the masters of their own destiny. They have lost their independence and their freedom to go and do as they wish. They must admit that they are no longer competent. They must learn to ask for help and rely on others. It can be a tragedy for many and a hardship for most. This chapter will help readers assess whether this step is necessary, and how to handle the situation with thoughtfulness, respect, and sensitivity.

As we grow older, we begin to lose physical strength and emotional security. We become more vulnerable to predators, who might target us specifically because they think we are weak. Chapter 10 arms you for the battle. You will learn how to handle con artists, avoid scams of every sort, combat telephone fraud, and prevent identity theft.

There is strength in numbers. Criminals know this and look for opportunities to catch us alone. They look for the solitary man or woman on the street, and then strike when we are least able to fight. But fight back we can—perhaps not with physical strength, but certainly with our brains and know-how. Chapter 11 will show you how to avoid dangerous situations in the first place, how to create a plan before venturing out, and how to deal with danger if and when it does occur.

Chapter 12 discusses some of the toughest issues we face as we grow older. Depression, fear, and grief are very real challenges for the aging, and the older we become, the greater the challenges become. If we live a long life, the likelihood of losing our loved ones increases. It is possible to experience the loss of friends and family members, a spouse, and even a child. These losses are hard to bear, and we all need help in coping with them.

Additionally, as we age, we begin to lose our faculties—sight, hearing, and strength. As a result, fear may become a more than occasional guest, and the issues it brings are varied and multifaceted. We fear being alone, but we also fear being a burden on anyone. We fear not being able to take care of ourselves, but we fear being taken advantage of by others. We fear change, but we also fear being left behind.

Growing older can be difficult for various reasons at every age. However, growing *old* can be terrifying. Chapter 12 addresses the issues that can make the last third of our life sad and sometimes even debilitating. There are sound suggestions, excellent resources, and clear-cut strategies for coping with whatever challenges we are called on to handle.

The final chapter discusses hope. Sometimes we forget that there *are* benefits to growing older. Because we have lived long enough to learn some important lessons, we are in the unique position of always being the best teacher in the room. We have lived long enough to see how life turns out. We have been allowed the privilege of watching our children and even grandchildren grow up, get launched, and forge their own ways in life. We have seen the fruits of our work change individuals and society, and we are able to live life more freely—without all the encumbrances of social dictate—but with greater honesty and more candor. Older people have earned the right to think and say what they wish without fear of reprisal. It truly is a unique position to be in.

Additionally, this chapter addresses gratitude for the opportunity to take care of those who are aging in our family. The benefits are numerous, as we have a chance to mend bridges and to say "I'm sorry," "thank you," and "I have always loved you." What a gift this time can be! There is also the satisfaction of knowing you have done what is right and good for a loved one.

*Living Agelessly* is a comprehensive guide for maintaining health and fitness as we approach mid-life and beyond. It is also filled with useful information for people just entering the retirement years, who might be taking care of their aging parents at the same time that they are devoting time and resources to their grandchildren. *Living Agelessly* can help older retirees—and those caring for them—take control of the more difficult aspects of growing older, including the potential for victimization and depression. Finally, *Living Agelessly* gives us hope and the tools to age with style and grace.

# Part I

## Recipe for Health and Fitness

# Aging Gracefully

*The Power of the Mind–Body–Spirit Connection*

Dear Ageless:

I'm constantly accused of being negative. I began to really listen to myself and found that my critics were right. I'm in my 50s. Is it too late to change?

Wanting to be Positive

Dear Wanting to be Positive:

It's never too late to change, and there are good reasons for being motivated. A negative attitude is destructive on many levels. It affects how others feel about you, how you feel about yourself, and how you feel physically. Research shows that people with heart disease, America's number one killer, are 40 percent less likely to laugh than those of the same age without heart disease.

Although researchers don't know how a positive attitude contributes to a healthier heart, they do know that mental stress and negativity affects the protective barrier that lines the blood vessels. So, in addition to exercise, not smoking, and a low-fat diet, it's crucial to your good health to add regular doses of hearty laughter.

*Living in the past or spending too much time planning for the future can prevent you from appreciating the present. Begin a gratitude journal. Date each entry and list all that was good in your day. Find value in the small things—nature, silence, a delicious meal—and you will cherish that which is most important: your relationships, abilities, and contributions to others.*

*The happiest people are those who continue to discover and share their special gifts, who seek to learn new things, and who reach out to help others rather than focus on themselves.*

*"Conquer Your Critical Inner Voice: A Revolutionary Program to Counter Negative Thoughts" by Robert W. Firestone, Lisa Firestone, and Joyce Catlet is an excellent book for overcoming negative thoughts and working through self-imposed limitations that impact intimacy, career, and quality of life.*

*Being positive is a choice. Even if you don't feel upbeat, behave as if you do. Your mind and body will respond. Others will be drawn to your warmth and friendliness. You'll begin to feel valued and loved, and you'll want to treat others the same way. It becomes the loveliest of cycles.*

*Ageless*

Aging is a natural phenomenon that begins the moment we are born. Although we celebrate each new year, we begin to yearn to be another age almost immediately after blowing out the candles.

Twelve-year-olds want to be 16, so they can date and drive. Sixteen-year-olds want to be 18, so they'll be considered adults. Eighteen-year-olds want to be 21, so they can drink and be independent. Thirty-year-olds want to be 21 again, because 30 seems old, especially if they haven't achieved the goals they set for themselves. Forty-year-olds experience a mid-life crisis. Fifty-year-olds struggle with empty-nest syndrome and the depression that comes with knowing that over half their life is gone. Sixty-year-olds must reassess their value to the world, especially if they are forced from the workplace. Seventy-year-olds begin to lose their physical prowess, and 80-year-olds their mental acuity.

This deep unease about current age and the process of aging erodes self-esteem, creates insecurity, and negates happiness. Filtering experiences through such a negative lens taints even the loveliest of times. Because the hope is so great that another age will be better than the present one, most of us live in the future rather than value and enjoy the present. Planning for the future is fine, although even the "best laid plans" sometimes go awry. *We just can't live there.*

## THE POWER OF THE MIND

Aging successfully is all about *attitude.* Because life is an unfolding process, feelings—even the most horrific ones—are transient, so take care not to be led by them. Decide to be in charge. It's critical to put your feelings into perspective, change your thought patterns, and choose your actions and reactions. Take pride in the accomplishments of the past and consider them the foundation of the present. Then appreciate the present, warts and all, because without the hard times, we wouldn't recognize the joy.

Don't obsess about failures. It can result in depression and even debilitation. Evaluate failures, so that you can learn from them, but then let them go. This is a healthy habit that you can begin to develop and eventually embrace, although in the beginning you might not think it's possible. Each time a negative thought comes to mind, choose to replace it with one that's positive. Have at your fingertips index cards with quotes, scriptures, or excerpts from books that inspire, uplift, and regenerate your thought process.

Words are powerful. Your words shape your memories, so choose your adjectives carefully when you describe your experiences, because they will be what you'll recall. Even if life has been difficult—and isn't that true for many of us?—searching for what is positive is crucial. An example of adopting a positive attitude might be: "I have survived so many challenges in the last 50 years and learned so much," rather than "My life has been one horrible problem after another."

You can alter your life by altering your attitude. Evidence is mounting that a positive attitude not only affects your quality of and contentment with life, but it also delays the aging process. For example, researchers at The University of Texas conducted a seven-year experiment with more than 1,500 relatively healthy people to assess whether there was a link between emotions and the onset of frailty.

They reported in the *Journal of Psychology and Aging* that, although genes and physical health play a role in aging, "Those people who had a positive outlook on life were significantly less likely to become frail than those who were more pessimistic." They speculated that positive emotions may directly affect the quality of health by altering the chemical balance of the body.

"I believe that there is a connection between mind and body," said lead researcher Dr. Glenn Ostir, "and that our thoughts and attitudes/emotions affect physical functioning and over-all health, whether through direct mechanisms like immune function or indirect mechanisms like social support networks."

Scientific evidence even suggests that a positive attitude can lengthen life. In a study of 660 people over 50 (338 men and 322 women), Yale University Associate Professor Becca Levy found that those with positive perceptions of aging lived 7.5 years longer than people with negative perceptions of getting older. She suggests, "This is a critical finding, as medical achievements in the area of longevity are generally considered a success when they extend life by 1–2 years. The implications of attitude elongating life by 7 years are extraordinary."

"Stereotypes of aging are probably internalized in childhood or adulthood, and are carried through into old age," Levy wrote in the *Journal of Personality and Social Psychology*. "I think older adults can think about ways to question some of those negative stereotypes that they encounter in everyday life, and that there is reason to believe that may have a positive impact over time."

Negative stereotypes of aging can also be countered by copying positive role models. Many active older people exude an optimistic attitude, attain goals, and forge ahead successfully, despite what society suggests about their age. They refuse to be told they can't do something, and they are a force to be reckoned with—and we would do well to emulate their attitude and behavior.

Developing a positive attitude is a matter of choice. Begin with listening to your internal dialogue. How much of it is negative? Do you tell yourself, "I'm not good enough," or "There's no way I can do that"? You may be shocked at the number of thoughts during just one hour that feed your insecurities and fears, and raise your stress level.

These destructive thoughts affect your body, your mood, your behavior, and your choices—every aspect of your life. When your internal dialogue is negative, your body releases stress hormones. Cardiovascular disease appears to be caused in part by the continuous production of stress hormones.

When the constant message in your head is, "I can't," in all likelihood, you won't forge ahead, you won't take risks, and you won't succeed. In many cases, you won't even *try*. Your own thoughts will have altered your behavior, limited your choices, and sabotaged your happiness.

It's never too late to change, and you can take steps to be more positive, including:

▶ *Begin by rewording the negative thoughts in your internal dialogue.* Irene Segal in her book *Just Coach It* suggests the following positive affirmations (She calls it self talk.):
  - I will think of myself as successful!
  - I will have positive expectations for everything I do!
  - I will remind myself of past successes!
  - I will not dwell on failures; I just will not repeat them!
  - I will surround myself with positive people and ideas!

    — I will keep trying until I achieve the results I want!

▶ *Stop listening to your inner critic.* It creates self-doubt, depression, and anger. This is the reason we are negative about ourselves and others. According to Segal, "When we listen to that inner critic, we are actually causing a separation from others, and separation from the best part of ourselves."

▶ *Be kinder to yourself and more compassionate.* An example might be choosing to focus on what you completed, rather than berating yourself for what you didn't finish during a given day. When you truly accept and love who you are—and don't succumb in a momentary situation to whatever transient feelings occur—you will be able to tap into your best professional and personal self.

▶ *Be forgiving of others.* When we're self-critical, we also tend to be critical of others when they don't do what we want. Our inner critic causes us to try and control and manipulate others. These efforts ultimately end in alienation.

▶ *Lighten up!* Decide what is really important in your life and why. Then choose your passions and laugh about the rest. Create humor in your life. If you're down, watch a comedy on film or television, read some jokes, or call someone who makes you belly laugh. You'll elevate your mood and burn some calories.

▶ *Get into the habit of smiling.* When you smile at others, it's an invitation to be treated lovingly, even on the telephone. The other person can "hear" your smile, and it can soften the most difficult conversations. So, even if you don't feel like it, smiling will encourage positive things to happen in your life, and soon you will be smiling because you have something to smile about.

▶ *Improve your diet,* increase your level of activity (increases endorphins, those feel-good hormones), and sleep more soundly.

▶ *Exercise your brain.* Play word games, keep up with current events, learn how to use a computer, and take a class. You will feel sharp, in the loop, more interesting, and powerful. Even small changes will increase your confidence level.

▶ *Decide what you love to do* and delegate or eliminate from your life the activities that do not agree with your decisions.

▶ *Choose to participate in pleasurable activities.* Go to the theater, concerts, or museums, take baths to reduce stress, read a good book, listen to music at home, and reconnect with old friends.

▶ *Become more spiritual.* People who attend religious services or are otherwise spiritually engaged, practice their beliefs, and relate to other believers, appear to live longer and more satisfying lives. Meditation and prayer also seem to be extraordinarily effective in reducing stress and increasing wellness.

▶ *Help others.* One of the best remedies for not obsessing about your own concerns is to focus on others. It helps with perspective and redirection, and just makes us feel good. Volunteer at your local hospital or read to the blind, run errands for an aging neighbor, deliver meals to someone who is housebound, become a foster grandparent to a child, or mentor a teenager. Working with kids will make *you* feel younger, too.

▶ *Find ways to love and be loved.* Communicating your feelings about difficulties minimizes their seeming enormity and power, and allows for new perspective. Holding in your feelings results in stress and frustration, withdrawal, and alienation from others. Caring about and sharing with friends and family alleviates feelings of depression and loneliness.

The one absolute in life is that we will all age and eventually die. The process begins the moment we're conceived, but the choice for how we handle this reality is one that we make from moment to moment. We may not be able to control the circumstances of our life (family, country of origin, genetics, and innate talent), but we *can* control our reaction to our circumstances.

## The Power of the Body

There is no question that a healthy diet, regular exercise, and eight hours of sleep are critical for the body to heal and rejuvenate itself. When you care properly for your body, you will be able to face the day with energy and the ability to complete tasks.

Even if all our physical needs are met, however, our energy will be drained and our ability to complete tasks compromised if we're struggling emotionally.

Important options are available—psychiatrists can prescribe drugs that may alleviate symptoms, psychologists can guide effective talk therapy, and counselors use techniques that can help educate us and change our behavior. Anyone who suffers with emotional problems should seek help in the same way they would for a physical ailment. Just like a physical disorder, an emotional disorder can worsen if left unattended, or improve with treatment.

▶ *Begin by having a check-up*, so that any physical component to your problem can be ruled out. Get referrals from your physician for appropriate professionals whom you might decide to interview.

▶ *Discuss your problem with people you trust*. Finding out that others share a similar struggle can alleviate some of the associated fear and isolation.

▶ *Ask your confidantes for the names of professionals who helped them resolve their issues*. Then set up interviews (yes . . . with doctors and other health care providers, too). Develop your list of questions before the conversation. Interviewing (which can be done on the telephone) allows you to determine if the philosophy and style of the person with whom you will be working makes you feel comfortable. If not, choose a different professional. If the health care provider is unwilling to be interviewed, that person is also not the professional for you.

▶ *Always get a second opinion* when you must make a serious decision about your health, and do not feel strange in telling your doctor that you intend to do so. Good doctors will encourage you to seek another doctor's advice or opinion. It's important to have a fresh perspective, and someone else to read your tests, X-rays, and charts. This policy reduces the risk of mistakes as well.

▶ *Know that some doctors refuse to give a second opinion.* Their hesitation is in possibly being in conflict with a colleague. It is not necessary to say at the onset that you are seeking another opinion. It's better, anyway, to allow the second doctor complete objectivity.

▶ *If the diagnosis is severe, ask for retesting.* Sometimes, labs make errors, and even another doctor won't catch it because he will be reading erroneous results.

▶ *Be sure to get a yearly exam* by both your physician and your gynecologist, if you are a woman. A regular assessment by your doctor will catch changes in your body that you may not have noticed because they have evolved slowly.

▶ *Take medicine as prescribed, and finish all antibiotics.* Resistance to antibiotics can result if you don't finish your medications as prescribed. If you have an adverse reaction—such as hives, lethargy, or disorientation—contact your doctor immediately.

▶ *Make sure your doctor knows all the medications you are taking* in order to avoid the danger that can come with polypharmacy (mixing of medications). Keep a list of all your medications, their dosages, and how often you take them on your refrigerator for paramedics, who may have to treat you in your home.

▶ *Keep a list of all your medications in your wallet.* You will have the list when your doctor asks you for an update, and it will also be available if you need emergency treatment, but, for whatever reason, you cannot communicate with hospital attendants.

▶ *If possible, consider getting all your prescriptions from one pharmacy.* The pharmacist can be of enormous help in identifying the danger that comes with polypharmacy, and in explaining potential problems that may come with mixing your particular medications.

In addition to conventional medical approaches to the resolution of your emotional or physical disorders, you can consider complementary and alternative medicine (CAM). Of course, you should *always* begin with a complete examination and evaluation by your physician or psychiatrist.

The fields of science and medicine recognize their limitations, and there has been an increasing acceptance of a holistic approach to good health. Over the last two decades, interest has grown in treating the whole person with what some consider more "natural" treatments.

This change in attitude began for a number of reasons, including severely adverse reactions to commonly used drugs, the availability to lay people of information about disease and disorders, and more astute and demanding consumers, who now know what physicians have known for a long time: The body is a living thing with the ability to heal itself, and conventional medical care must integrate a more natural approach that includes medicines that offer safe and effective ways to treat the individual without side effects.

*Before beginning any practice that fits under the category of complementary medicine, it is critical that you see your physician, discuss any treatment you're contemplating, and consider these efforts to be an adjunct to conventional therapies that have been prescribed for your symptoms. Never use alternative therapies instead of conventional therapies—that's why the word "complementary" is preferred.*

Before beginning any practice that fits under the category of complementary medicine, it is critical that you see your physician, discuss any treatment you're contemplating, and consider these efforts to be an adjunct to conventional therapies that have been prescribed for your symptoms. Never use alternative therapies instead of conventional therapies—that's why the word "complementary" is preferred.

Practitioners of *naturopathic medicine* use a holistic approach with their patients. They prefer not to use synthetic drugs or invasive surgery, although practitioners from accredited schools are trained to use diagnostic tools such as blood tests and magnetic resonance imaging (MRI). Be sure your practitioner is licensed to practice under the laws of the state where you live, and be aware that good practitioners are willing to refer patients to a medical doctor when necessary.

Naturopathy includes various modalities (treatment types):

- *Clinical nutrition and life style changes*—the assessment of risk factors associated with the environment and life choices
- *Herbal medicine*—the use of food and herbs as therapy
- *Hygiene*—the use of hydrotherapy—hot and cold water, sauna, and steam
- *Physical manipulation*—bone alignment similar to osteopathic and chiropractic adjustments, although you must take great care in choosing your practitioner. If not done properly, dramatic and permanent damage can result.
- *Traditional Chinese medicine*—based on the belief that good health can be achieved when a balance is present between the body's biochemistry, biomechanics, and emotional predisposition.
- *Acupuncture*—best-known technique associated with traditional Chinese medicine and recommended by the World Health Organization for the treatment of a number of conditions. The best available evidence is for the use of acupuncture in the management of pain. Acupuncture and acupressure therapies are considered part of the broader concept of *energy medicine*, which is also based on the theory that the body has meridians (energy pathways) that can be blocked or disrupted. Acupuncturists believe that illness, both physical and emotional, results, in part, from blockages or disturbances in the energy flow in the body. Acupuncture and acupressure are forms of stimulating specific "points" along the meridians to correct imbalances. Needles are used in acupuncture whereas the points are manually stimulated in acupressure.
- *Emotional freedom techniques (EFT)*—the practice of "psychological acupressure" based on the same energy meridians used in traditional

acupuncture; instead of needles being placed strategically along the meridians of the body, tapping is used to stimulate trigger points.

▶ *Meditation*—an ancient mind–body practice that can increase physical relaxation and psychological balance. It is a conscious mental process that causes physiologic changes that, in turn, induce a relaxation response. Practitioners claim relief from a variety of ailments, including pain, anxiety, depression, stress, and insomnia, resulting in an overall improvement in wellness. Most types of meditation have several elements in common, including the preference for a quiet location, a specific posture that varies depending on the type of mediation, and focused attention on an object, breath, or *mantra*, which is a word or phrase usually related to a spiritual concept; for example, "Om."

## The Power of the Spirit

For thousands of years, people of nearly every faith have believed that an attitude of prayerfulness, caring, and compassion for those in need sets the stage for healing.

Recent scientific studies show that prayer and meditation can be powerful medicine—positively affecting high blood pressure, heart attacks, headaches, and anxiety. They inhibit the hormones that flow from the adrenal glands in response to stress. In addition to drugs, surgery, and other conventional therapies, prayer and meditation are considered a vital component to recovery from surgery, illness, and disease.

Seniors often become depressed when they are no longer able to worship as they once did. Sometimes they can no longer attend services because of a physical disability or a logistical issue, such as a lack of transportation. Find out whether someone at your place of worship or in your neighborhood needs help getting to services.

If they are content to stay home—and they are open to it—take some aspect of their preferred religious service to them. If they find it comforting and pleasurable, play songs of worship when you visit and leave behind a compilation of favorites on CD or cassette tape. Ask permission to invite their spiritual leader to accompany you on a visit.

Following basic guidelines for a more spiritual life can contribute to the reduction of stress and create a more positive outlook on life. Spirituality teaches us:

- ▶ *To have faith in something greater than ourselves.* When we relinquish worry and control, we feel more peaceful about life. The reality is that worry doesn't produce anything of value. It's very much like being in a rocking chair—you're constantly moving, but it doesn't get you anywhere.
- ▶ *To relinquish manipulation.* Controlling our environment, and the people in it, is an illusion. The only true control we can exercise is over ourselves, and sometimes we're not particularly successful at that! When we loosen our stranglehold on the serious issues in our life, we often find peace even in the midst of the storm.
- ▶ *To give to the less fortunate.* This helps on several levels besides the obvious one. The body releases endorphins (the "feel-good" hormones), so we actually feel better physically and emotionally when we are giving to others. Investing in others is also a distraction from our own problems, which are often minimized when we see firsthand the challenges and even greater hardships that others face. We can't worry so much about ourselves when we are busy helping others who are hurting more.
- ▶ *To accept the past and not dwell on the mistakes we made.* Berating ourselves for what we cannot change drains us of energy and time that could be spent more constructively. We cannot change what's happened, and if we continue to immerse ourselves in it, we are guaranteed a life of regret rather than one of pride, pleasure, and purpose.
- ▶ *To forgive others their transgressions.* This is perhaps the hardest precept of all, but the most freeing. Not forgiving someone is

comparable to swallowing poison yourself, and then waiting for the person you can't forgive to die. Often, the person you can't forgive doesn't even know you're still angry, and as long as you do not forgive, you are allowing that person to have control over your life. Forgiving others is not a gift to the person we are forgiving, but a gift to ourselves. It alleviates the bitterness that can shroud our life and eradicates the poison that can destroy it.

▶ *To be grateful.* If you are thankful for the gifts in your life, you will force yourself to be positive. Others will be attracted to your optimistic nature, and your attitude will be contagious. Look for goodness, and you will find it.

▶ *To surround yourself with like-minded people.* You may not be able to choose your family members, but you can choose those with whom you will spend your time. Select people who encourage your efforts and inspire you to be your best self.

▶ *To invest in others.* Give of yourself, and when you need help—and we all do from time to time—others will invest in you.

The scientific and medical communities recognize the power of the mind–body–spirit connection to heal or harm. It's undeniable that this connection can create the environment for illness or a state of wellness, both physically and psychologically.

Medical treatment can be viewed as a three-legged stool comprised of medical and surgical management, pharmaceutical and complementary medicine, and self-care that includes nutrition, exercise, spirituality, and relaxation for enjoyment and stress reduction.

Using multiple approaches can improve your quality of life and the possibility for physical and emotional health. Many of these approaches are patient-friendly as well. Anyone can learn cost-effective ways to contribute to their own healing.

# Food as Potent Medicine

*Nutrition for a Zestful Life*

*Dear Ageless:*

*What's all the fuss about fats in our diet? I keep hearing and reading that oils containing omega-3 polyunsaturated fat can prevent disease. True or not?*

*The Family Cook*

*Dear Family Cook:*

*The power of food to prevent disease is undeniable, and our decisions regarding it are the primary cause for how we feel and operate. In order to achieve and/or maintain good health, we need to understand the four critical components of a healthy diet: protein, carbohydrates, water, and fat. The topic of fat intake seems to be the most confusing for many people.*

*Scientific studies show that the type of fat we consume (saturated, monounsaturated, or polyunsaturated) alters compounds in our bodies that affect our mental, emotional, and physical well-being—including the brain, heart, cell, immune, and vision function.*

Omega-3 fatty acids are considered "essential" because they are crucial to cell structure and body function, but they are not produced by the body. They must be supplied by including in your diet such foods as cold-water fish (wild salmon, mackerel, sardines, and fresh tuna), fish oil, cod liver oil, dark green leafy vegetables, walnuts, flax seeds, and flax oil. "The Omega Plan: The Medically Proven Diet That Restores Your Body's Essential Nutritional Balance" by Dr. Artemis Simopoulos contains extensive information on this subject.

According to the American Heart Association, a diet rich in omega-3 fatty acids helps cut the risk of cardiovascular disease; helps prevent diseases such as diabetes, rheumatoid arthritis, and psoriasis; and may improve some aspects of mental health, such as depression.

The challenge is getting enough omega-3-containing fats from food sources; fish needs to be consumed at least twice a week. You may need to supplement your diet, but the additional benefits are many. They include reducing blood pressure and systemic (whole body) inflammation (reducing joint aches); improving the composition and strength of cell membranes (preventing stiffness); reducing triglyceride and cholesterol levels; reducing plaque on the walls of arteries (improving heart health); preventing some cancers (breast, colon, and stomach); nourishing the hair, skin, and nails; improving metabolism (leading to weight reduction), alleviating psoriasis; and improving memory, learning, and mental health.

Researchers exploring possible links between diet and mental illness have found that increasing our consumption of certain "good" fats may also improve the symptoms of psychiatric illnesses, including depression, bipolar disorder, and even schizophrenia. For additional information visit the National Institutes of Health at www.nih.gov, or www.nlm.nih.gov.

Ageless

We have become a society that hotly pursues the "quick fix" and indiscriminately takes a variety of drugs to solve our ailments. The problems of prescription abuse and mixing medications, which can result in adverse interactions, are on the rise, and seniors who have multiple health issues are particularly vulnerable.

Until recently, we've looked askance at the advice of doctors who have a "holistic" approach and recommend the use of "natural" remedies to achieve good health. We've ignored our grandmothers, too, who—through experience—promoted one food or another for wellness. This might have included chicken soup for colds, carrots for good vision, and an apple a day—all of which are clichés that are actually good advice. The tide is changing, however, and the level of respect for how food can affect the body as powerfully as prescribed medication is increasing.

For over 4,000 years, healers and physicians have used food as a critical part of their prescription for good health and disease prevention. In our quest to "enjoy" the dining experience (however that might be defined) or "just get meals over with" (there really are people who eat only because they're supposed to), many of us have forgotten how critical food really is to every aspect of our existence.

A lifestyle that includes regular health care, medicine to treat illness, exercise, and a good diet is the prescription for a long and healthy life.

For most of us, particularly in North America, where food of every sort is widely available and obesity is on the rise among adults and children, what sounds or looks good is generally the guiding principle for food choice. What's easy and fast is another consideration. We've lost sight of the principle of "food as medicine," which is critical for sustaining life and necessary for optimal functioning.

Although we may not be able to control a number of factors in our lives—genetic make-up, family of origin, environment, and the behavior of others—we can and must exercise control over what we do and do not eat. What we feed our "engine" each day determines how well we "run."

## Proteins Beef Up Good Health

Protein is a critical component of every cell in the body. Protein is a *macronutrient*, meaning that it is critical to the body in substantial amounts. It's used to build and repair tissue, including bones, muscles, cartilage, skin, and blood.

Unlike the other three macronutrients—carbohydrates, fats, and water—the body does not store protein, so there is no easily available reservoir from which to draw. Protein must be consumed daily to maintain physical strength, repair muscle, and produce energy. However, we don't need as much protein in our diets as you might suppose.

Adults generally need 60 grams of protein per day, which should represent 10–15 percent of their total caloric intake. The American Heart Association recommends the following:

- ▶ Teenage boys and active men can get all the protein they need from three daily servings that total 7 ounces.
- ▶ Older children, teen-aged girls, active women, and most men need two daily servings that total 6 ounces.
- ▶ Children age 2–6, most women, and some older people need two daily servings that total 5 ounces.

The challenge is to create a protein-rich diet that does not increase the risk of cardiovascular disease, which can result from too much of the saturated fat found in animal foods. A protein-rich diet derived from both animal and plant sources—such as beans, nuts, seeds, and a number of grains—can decrease the risk of cardiovascular disease by about 20 percent. Alternatives to red meat include:

- ▶ *Fish* has less fat than red meat and offers heart-healthy omega-3 fatty acids.
- ▶ *Poultry* is excellent, and you can eliminate most of the saturated fat by removing the skin.

- ▶ *Beans* contain more protein than any other vegetable. They also contain fiber that helps you feel full for hours.
- ▶ *Nuts* of various types give you the same amount of protein as meat—for example, 1 ounce of almonds gives you 6 grams of protein, almost as much as 1 ounce of steak—and nuts are a source of healthier fats.
- ▶ *Whole grains*—such as those in a slice of whole wheat bread—give you 3 grams of protein, plus valuable fiber.
- ▶ *Soy* offers a high-protein alternative without saturated fat or cholesterol. Soy beans are the only beans considered to be a complete protein, because they contain all eight essential amino acids.
- ▶ *Eggs* are one of the most nutritious sources of protein. They are low in calories, relatively low in saturated fat, and a good source of vitamins.

## Carbohydrates Sweeten the Pot

Carbohydrates ("carbs") are critical to our well-being, but they have been criticized as the major component of unhealthy diets. Modern thinking has dubbed the carb the "obesity culprit," and eliminated it from numerous weight loss strategies. This can be dangerous. Carbs don't just make us feel energetic; they are a primary energy source for our bodies, and they supply vitamins and minerals that are critical to good health.

There are two types of carbohydrates—*simple* and *complex*. Both are converted into glucose and are either used immediately as an energy source or stored for later use.

Simple carbohydrates are broken down the most rapidly by our bodies; they are the quickest source of energy. They are found in fruits (fructose), sugars (sucrose), and milk (lactose).

Complex carbohydrates are broken down more slowly to provide longer-term energy. They are found as starches in breads and pastas; in grains, such as corn, rice, rye, and other grains besides wheat; in root vegetables, such as potatoes and carrots; and in beans. Complex carbohydrates are also a good source of the dietary fiber that is critical for binding and eliminating cholesterol, cleansing the digestive tract, preventing constipation and hemorrhoids, and reducing the risk of colon cancer.

Your diet should contain 30 mg or more a day of fiber, and 40–50 percent of our caloric intake should be made up of carbohydrates. You should not eat much more than this amount because the excess will be stored as fat.

## WATER KEEPS US FLUSH

We don't generally think of water as one of the four main nutrients, but, in fact, it's one of the most critical. Water is necessary for all circulatory, digestive, absorption, and excretory functions. It transports nutrients and waste products into and out of cells, helps maintain proper body temperature, and affects our energy level. Water prevents bacterial, viral, and fungal infections by flushing out the harmful impurities and toxins in our bodies.

We often replace water almost completely with coffee, tea, milk, juice, sodas, and even alcohol. With so many options, some people never add water to the list of beverages they drink. This is a *huge* mistake, and dehydration—which becomes an increasingly greater problem as we grow older—is not the only consequence.

Water acts as a lubricant for the tissues in our bodies—much like the oil in our car. We would never consider driving without proper lubrication, but some of us take in too little water to operate properly. Chronic dehydration may be the root cause of a variety of diseases, including bladder and kidney infections, arthritis, and chronic constipation, which can result in problems such as hemorrhoids.

We sometimes confuse hunger with thirst. See if drinking a glass of water satisfies you before opening the refrigerator. It's an excellent appetite suppressant, and it's effective in promoting the metabolism and elimination of stored fat.

Drink sips of water throughout the day, as your body can only process about 8 ounces per hour unless you're exercising. Be sure to increase water intake before, during, and after exercise. Eight 8-ounce glasses every day is sufficient for optimal health.

## FATS: WHAT'S THE SKINNY?

Fats are essential to your body. They provide energy, support cell growth, help protect your organs, and keep your body warm. Fats also help your body absorb some nutrients, and they are the basis for making the hormones crucial to your body's normal functioning.

Fats are comprised of building blocks called *essential fatty acids*. There are three types: saturated, polyunsaturated, and monounsaturated.

*Saturated* fatty acids are found mostly in animal products, such as meat and whole milk. Butter and lard are also high in saturated fatty acids. Too much saturated fat can promote coronary artery disease and raise blood cholesterol, including *low density lipoproteins* (LDLs). It can be the culprit for making the sticky, yellow deposit called *plaque* that attaches to artery walls, thereby reducing the flow of blood to the heart (resulting in cardiovascular disease) and the brain (resulting in a stroke).

Saturated fats are found in dairy products, including whole milk, cream, and cheese; hydrogenated vegetable shortening; and some oils—including coconut and palm kernel oils. Saturated fats are also found in animal products, including beef, pork, ham, veal, and lamb. As a rule of thumb, the more solid the food, the more saturated the fat.

*Polyunsaturated* fats are a good source of the essential fatty acids, which can't be manufactured by the body but are necessary for good health. This type of fat is found in salmon, mackerel, herring, sardines, tuna, and other deep-sea fish. Polyunsaturated fats include the omega-

3 fats, which are so important to heart and liver health because they fight inflammation and lower triglycerides.

Polyunsaturated fats are also found in vegetable and nut oils, including corn, soybean, flaxseed, canola, safflower, sunflower, walnuts, and pecans. These are all good sources of omega-6 fats, which can reduce or prevent the inflammation that causes premature aging.

*Monounsaturated* fats are considered the healthiest type of fat because they lower low-density lipoprotein (LDL; "bad" cholesterol) levels and raise high-density lipoprotein (HDL; "good" cholesterol). They come from the fruits and oils of olives, avocados, canola, apricots, almonds, and peanuts. The best of these oils are those that are "cold pressed," not heat processed, because heat changes the chemical structure of even healthy polyunsaturated oils into *trans-fat*—which is considered the most dangerous type of fat.

Oils are a better choice for cooking, as well, because they remain stable at higher temperatures and don't become rancid or break down into trans-fats. Coconut, grapeseed, and olive oil are the best oils for sautéing.

The American Heart Association recommendations for an overall healthy diet and lifestyle that will combat heart disease includes eating less than 7 percent of our total daily calories as saturated fats and less than 1 percent as trans-fats. In practical terms, this means eating a diet containing a variety of fruits, vegetables, and grain products (especially whole grains), fat-free and low-fat dairy products, legumes, poultry, lean meats, and fish (preferably oily fish) at least twice a week.

Here are guidelines for choosing good fats:

► *Read the ingredients listed on food labels.* If you find the words "hydrogenated" or "partially hydrogenated" on the list, don't buy the product. If you already have these products in your kitchen, throw them away.
► *Do not eat trans-fats.* Although food manufacturers are beginning to replace trans-fat in their products, be wary of other artificial

ingredients that may have been added to keep the original taste and/or consistency. Check before buying processed foods, because they tend to be loaded with trans-fats, and avoid fast food restaurants that use trans-fats in cooking (some fast food chains are now addressing this issue).

▶ *Limit saturated fats* to less than 7 percent of the total calories in your diet.

▶ *Eat real, natural fat and cholesterol* in moderate amounts as part of every meal. Snack on olives, sardines, nuts, and nut butters, and eat moderate amounts of protein—a great source of natural fat—at each meal to sustain energy, minimize blood sugar spikes, and feel fuller all day.

▶ *Use only cold-pressed oils*, and keep cooking oils in the refrigerator to avoid rancidity. Olive and grapeseed oils are the most stable for cooking over moderate heat. Avoid cooking over high heat because the temperature can change even good fat into *trans-fat.*

Buy only the best quality dairy products from reliable sources—preferably organic, if you can afford the higher prices. Growth hormones, antibiotics, and environmental toxins, such as pesticides and heavy metals, accumulate in the fat cells of animals. When we ingest their milk or meat, we are eating high levels of these toxins. Our natural response is low-grade inflammation, which is a good thing, sometimes, because it fights substances that are foreign and harmful in our body. However, inflammation is bad for our bodies when it is chronic. See *The Anti-Inflammation Diet and Recipe Book* by Jessica K. Black for more information on this subject.

Try the suggestions in Table 2-1, from the American Heart Association, to substitute healthy alternatives in your diet.

Taking care of your body throughout your lifetime—by eating the proper foods in the proper amounts—can go a long way to assuring that you will be healthy and happy as you get older. Make the investment in yourself right now, no matter what age you are.

**TABLE 2.1** *Substituting Ingredients*

| When recipe calls for... | Use this instead... |
| --- | --- |
| Whole milk (1 cup) | 1 cup fat-free or low-fat milk, plus 1 tablespoon of liquid vegetable oil |
| Heavy cream (1 cup) | 1 cup evaporated skim milk or 1/2 cup low-fat yogurt and 1/2 cup plain low-fat unsalted cottage cheese |
| Sour cream | Low-fat unsalted cottage cheese plus low-fat or fat-free yogurt; or just use fat-free sour cream, which is also available |
| Cream cheese | 4 tablespoons soft margarine (low in saturated fat and 0 grams *trans-fat*) blended with 1 cup dry, unsalted low-fat cottage cheese; add a small amount of fat-free milk if needed |
| Butter (1 tablespoon) | 1 tablespoon soft margarine (low in saturated fat and 0 grams *trans-fat*) or 3/4 tablespoon liquid vegetable oil |
| Egg (2 per week) | 2 egg whites; or choose a commercially made, cholesterol-free egg substitute (1/4 cup) |
| Unsweetened baking chocolate (1 ounce) | 3 tablespoons unsweetened cocoa powder or carob powder plus 1 tablespoon vegetable oil or soft margarine; carob is sweeter than cocoa, so reduce the sugar. |

# Spice Up Your Diet

*Antioxidants for an Anti-Aging Lifestyle*

*Dear Ageless:*

*I keep hearing about the health benefits of cooking with spices. It seems they cure everything from the deadliest cancers to an ailing sex life. Should I be spicing it up?*

*Dull in the Kitchen*

*Dear Dull:*

*For centuries, our ancestors considered spices and herbs to be the answer to many medical problems. Over time, spices became more respected for their culinary enhancements than for their medicinal value, but recent studies are demonstrating their healing properties.*

*Experts don't suggest substituting spices (plant bark, root, bud, or berry) or herbs (herbaceous plant leaves) for a healthy, well-balanced diet, and warn that consuming too much of any food additive can be risky, but they do advocate the use of spices for diet diversification and boosting the health value of a meal.*

*Use fresh instead of processed spices and herbs whenever possible, because they contain higher levels of antioxidants. Buy spices whole and grind them just before use, crush dried leaves or herbs, and use whole sprigs in long-cooking dishes for maximum benefit. Add sprigs of oregano or rosemary to vegetable, rice, and pasta cooking water. Herbal teas (sage, rosemary, thyme, oregano, peppermint, spearmint) retain their antioxidant properties even after a 30-minute boiling time.*

*Ageless*

The American Spice Trade Association believes that people began to use spices for medicinal purposes and cooking as early as 50,000 BCE. Throughout history, spices were considered so valuable that they became a form of currency that sent explorers around the world. Marco Polo opened up the Spice Route to China; Christopher Columbus found America during his search for new spice sources; Britain occupied India, in part, to control its spice and tea trade; and Magellan circumnavigated the globe and returned with enough spices to finance the entire voyage. In those days, spices created wealth. Today, they can help prevent disease and create health.

Some of the more common uses of herbs and spices are:

▶ Peppermint has been used to treat gastric and digestive disorders, tension, and insomnia.
▶ Mustard may relieve respiratory problems.
▶ Cayenne pepper and Tabasco sauce are believed by some to increase the rate of metabolism and fat-burning ability by as much as 25 percent.
▶ Ginger inhibits the nausea and vomiting associated with morning or motion sickness.
▶ Allspice relieves indigestion and gas.
▶ Cinnamon (which you can buy in capsules) combats diarrhea, and is believed to enhance glucose metabolism and to kill bacteria and other microorganisms.

▶ Turmeric is believed to neutralize free radicals, protect against cancer, and may be a natural anti-inflammatory agent.

▶ Cumin is considered by some to be a protective agent against the development of cancer.

▶ Garlic may decrease blood pressure, appears to be a natural antibiotic, and may be beneficial in the treatment of diabetes.

▶ Oregano has three to twenty times the antioxidant activity of other herbs.

Consult your physician before making any dietary changes, and never substitute spices or herbal supplements for prescribed medication. See *The Green Pharmacy* by Dr. James Duke and *Spices of Life* and *A Spoonful of Ginger* by Nina Simonds to learn recipes for a healthy lifestyle.

## ANTIOXIDANTS

In addition to making foods tastier, spices are powerful antioxidants. What are antioxidants, and what makes them so important?

*Oxidation* damage is closely linked to the formation of *free radicals*, which are both a normal product of our body's metabolism and the cause of damage in various cells. Aging, stress, and environmental factors increase the number of free radicals in the body.

Free radicals are now considered to be a major factor in the development of many degenerative diseases, including cancer, cardiovascular disease, cognitive impairment, Alzheimer's disease, immune dysfunction, cataracts, and macular degeneration.

*Antioxidants* are the body's defense mechanism against free radicals. Antioxidants stabilize free radicals before they can cause harm. As we grow older, the body's defense mechanism against free radicals becomes less effective at the same time that oxidative stress in the body becomes greater.

As a result, we need to supplement the body's production of antioxidants with those found in fresh fruits, vegetables, and spices.

## Antioxidants in Spices

Ounce for ounce, spices may have even more antioxidant compounds than fruits and vegetables. For example, as little as 1 gram (about ½ teaspoon) of cloves contains more dietary antioxidant than a half-cup serving of blueberries or cranberries, both of which are known for their high antioxidant levels. One-half teaspoon of dried oregano contains as much antioxidant as ½ cup of sweet potatoes.

In a U.S. Department of Agriculture (USDA) review of 39 herbs, researchers found that oregano, dill, thyme, and rosemary have some of the highest levels of cancer-fighting antioxidants. Turmeric, sage, cloves, ginger, and chili pepper may also help fight the disease. (As noted throughout this book, however, *never* use complementary approaches such as dietary strategies *instead* of standard medical therapies.)

Many fresh herbs contain such high levels of antioxidants that they are still quite potent after drying. This includes cloves, allspice, cinnamon, rosemary, thyme, marjoram, saffron, oregano, tarragon, and basil. The best fresh herbs are oregano, sage, peppermint, thyme, and marjoram.

Ginger, generally associated with Asian cooking, is not only a powerful cancer-fighting antioxidant, but it's believed by some to aid in preventing Alzheimer's disease. Ginger also helps significantly with motion and seasickness, and it can reduce the nausea and vomiting brought on by pregnancy. To calm the stomach, drink 1–2 ounces of steeped ginger root. Ginger also contains an inflammation-fighting substance called *gingerol*, which may help reduce joint pain throughout the body and improve function in people who have arthritis.

Garlic has long been considered to have antiviral, antifungal, and antibacterial properties, and it can contribute to lowering blood pressure. Some studies now suggest that it might also play a role in preventing or slowing cancer, particularly of the stomach and prostate. Fresh garlic is best used just after peeling, but it can be pressed into an oil or powder. The active ingredient in garlic, *allicin*, is destroyed within an hour of crushing, so garlic pills are worthless. Avoid eating garlic in excess, as it can cause an allergic reaction, dermatitis, or stomach disorders.

Curry is a mixture of spices used routinely in Indian and other South Asian cooking. A team from the University of California believes that turmeric, one of the spices in curry, may slow the advance of Alzheimer's. This theory may explain why far fewer villagers over age 65 (in a study conducted in India) have the disease when compared with their Western counterparts. See *The Spice Is Right: Easy Indian Cooking for Today* by Monica Bhide for more information.

## Antioxidants in Plant Form

A healthy diet that includes foods rich in antioxidants has the potential to delay the onset of many age-related diseases. Vitamins A, C, and E; carotene; selenium; and lycopene are food components that act as antioxidants. These substances are found in plant foods, including fruits, vegetables, and whole grains.

Foods rich in antioxidants often have distinctive hues—generally rich, dark colors; for example, the deep red of tomatoes, peppers, and cherries; the blue, purple, and black of berries and grapes; orange carrots and sweet potatoes; and yellow corn.

The American Heart Association recommends that adults should eat five or more servings a day of a variety of fruits and vegetables that are rich in antioxidants, including:

> *Foods rich in antioxidants often have distinctive hues— generally rich, dark colors; for example, the deep red of tomatoes, peppers, and cherries; the blue, purple, and black of berries and grapes; orange carrots and sweet potatoes; and yellow corn.*

▶ At least one serving of a vitamin A-rich fruit or vegetable a day
▶ At least one serving of a vitamin C-rich fruit or vegetable a day

▶ At least one serving of a high-fiber fruit or vegetable a day

▶ Several servings of cruciferous vegetables—such as broccoli, cauliflower, and Brussels sprouts—a week

Serving sizes of some common foods are:

▶ 1 medium fruit or ½ cup of small or cut-up fruit

▶ ¾ cup (180 milliliters) of 100 percent juice

▶ ¼ cup dried fruit

▶ ½ cup raw non-leafy or cooked vegetables

▶ 1 cup raw leafy vegetables (such as lettuce)

▶ ½ cup cooked beans or peas (such as lentils, pinto beans, and kidney beans)

Some fruits, vegetables, and beans may be powerful aids in controlling diabetes, decreasing the risk of Alzheimer's and heart disease, and slowing the growth of tumors.

## Antioxidants in Your Pantry

*Cranberry.* For centuries, people have been using cranberries to cure a variety of ailments, especially urinary tract infections (UTIs). Drinking cranberry juice may also be a helpful way to prevent a UTI, inhibit the stomach acid that can result in peptic ulcers, and fight free radicals.

*Pomegranate.* The pomegranate has the highest level of antioxidants of any fruit, and it's the most effective fruit juice for combating free radicals that may contribute to the development of various diseases associated with aging. It contains more than three times the antioxidant properties of red wine or green tea. In fact, one pomegranate provides 40 percent of an adult's recommended daily allowance of vitamin C. Pomegranate is also a rich source of folic acid and vitamins A and E.

*Chocolate.* Studies show that chocolate can lower high blood pressure, and it's a potent antioxidant. This is true only for dark chocolate,

**TABLE 3.1** *Health-promoting Foods*

| | |
|---|---|
| Carrots, apples, citrus, onions, broccoli, tea | Neutralizes free radicals that can damage cells and bolsters cellular antioxidant defenses |
| Kale, collards, corn spinach, citrus, eggs | Contributes to maintenance of healthy vision |
| Fresh and processed tomatoes | Contributes to prostate health |
| Grapes, berries, cherries | Bolsters cellular defenses and contributes to brain function |
| Tea, cocoa, chocolate, apples, grapes | Contributes to heart health |
| Cranberries, apples, strawberries, grapes, peanuts, cinnamon cocoa, wine | Contributes to heart and urinary tract health |
| Cauliflower, broccoli, kale cabbage, horseradish | Detoxifies unhealthy compounds and contributes to healthy immune function |
| Garlic, onions, leeks, scallions | Contributes to heart health and immune function |
| Whole grains and cereals | Reduces the risk of coronary heart disease, cancer, and diabetes |

however, not milk or white chocolate. Dark chocolate should not be eaten with milk, because it reduces the ability of the antioxidant to be absorbed by the body.

Cocoa—the plant from which chocolate is made—is taken through several steps to reduce its naturally pungent taste, especially in North America. The *flavonoids* in cocoa are the reason both for its pungent taste and its power as an antioxidant. The more that chocolate is processed, the more flavonoids are destroyed, and the less potent the chocolate is as an antioxidant.

The recommended dose of flavonoids is 250–1,000 milligrams a day. To contribute to this amount, consider using organic Central American cacao beans, which are more gently processed.

The USDA warns that the extra calories consumed from eating dark chocolate must be balanced by eating less of other things. "A 100-gram serving of Hershey's Special Dark Chocolate Bar™ has 531 calories. If you ate that much raw apple, you'd only take in 52 calories."

*Apple Cider Vinegar.* Some researchers contend that the beta-carotene in apple cider vinegar makes it an antioxidant that destroys the free radicals in the body that compromise the immune system, cause tissue mutation, and expedite aging.

> *The USDA warns that the extra calories consumed from eating dark chocolate must be balanced by eating less of other things. "A 100-gram serving of Hershey's Special Dark Chocolate Bar™ has 531 calories. If you ate that much raw apple, you'd only take in 52 calories."*

*Coffee.* We are a nation of coffee drinkers, but lately we've been on a rollercoaster ride as to whether it's good for us or not. We use coffee to wake us up in the morning, to enliven us when we're lethargic in the afternoon, and to lift our mood whenever necessary. Research suggests that it may also reduce the chances of getting asthma, type 2 diabetes, gallstones, and cirrhosis of the liver. It may even lower the risk of Parkinson's disease, colon cancer, and Alzheimer's disease.

According to Bennett Alan Weinberg, Ph.D. and Bonnie Bealer, the authors of *The World of Caffeine,* "The key is knowing what caffeine can do for you and how to use it effectively." Here are just some of its possible benefits:

- ▶ It improves your ability to think clearly and solve problems, and can temporarily raise your IQ.
- ▶ It increases your short-term memory and helps you concentrate.
- ▶ It's a powerful antioxidant.
- ▶ It improves your mood.

These possibilities seem to outweigh the increased heart rate and blood pressure that some coffee drinkers experience, particularly as drinking decaffeinated coffee can diminish those issues. The extra calories from added cream and sugar can also be a problem, so black is best unless you use skim milk instead of cream.

The National Coffee Association suggests the following power drink—a coffee banana smoothie that is a smart snack. Yogurt is a stellar source of calcium; the banana adds potassium; wheat germ supplies extra vitamin E; and coffee contributes some kick:

---

**"The Power Lift"**

Makes four 8-ounce servings

1½ cups brewed coffee, cold or at room temperature
2 6-ounce containers plain low-fat yogurt (1½ cups)
2 medium ripe bananas, peeled and sliced
3 to 4 ice cubes
2 tablespoons toasted wheat germ
2 tablespoons honey, or to taste

Place all ingredients in a blender container. Cover, and blend on high speed for 1 minute, or until smooth. Pour into 4 glasses. Serve immediately.

Per serving: Calories, 154; Protein, 6 grams; Carbohydrates, 30 grams; Fat, 2 grams; Cholesterol, 5 mg; Sodium, 63 mg.

---

## VITAMINS AND MINERALS

Often referred to as *micronutrients*, vitamins and minerals are essential to life, but needed in relatively small amounts compared with the four basic *macronutrients* (protein, carbohydrate, fat, and water).

Table 3.2 summarizes the vitamins you need to maximize health, and their best sources.

**TABLE 3.2** *Vitamins We Need for Good Health*

| | |
|---|---|
| Vitamin A | For healthy skin, eyes, bones, hair, and teeth<br>*Source: apricots, oatmeal, fortified dairy products* |
| Vitamin $B_1$ (Thiamine) | For a properly functioning nervous system and normal appetite<br>*Source: green beans, grains, milk* |
| Vitamin $B_2$ (Riboflavin) | Healthy skin and eyes<br>*Source: nuts, cheese, eggs* |
| Vitamin $B_3$ (Niacin) | Releases energy from foods to maintain skin, nervous system, and proper mental functioning<br>*Source: meat, yeast* |
| Vitamin $B_6$ | Helps to metabolize protein and fat in the function of red blood cells and hemoglobin synthesis<br>*Source: egg yolk, wheat germ* |
| Vitamin $B_{12}$ | Prevents anemia; necessary for healthy nervous system; involved in synthesis of genetic material (DNA)<br>*Source: liver, milk, eggs, fish* |
| Vitamin C | Important for bones, teeth, collagen, and blood vessel (capillaries) maintenance; enables iron absorption and red blood cell formation<br>*Source: oranges, lemons, limes, grapefruit* |
| Vitamin D | Aids the absorption and metabolism of calcium and phosphorus for strong bones and teeth<br>*Source: dairy products* |
| Vitamin E | Protects red blood cells, lipoproteins, cell membranes, fats, and vitamin A from destructive oxidation<br>*Source: wheat germ* |
| Vitamin K | Needed for proper blood clotting<br>*Source: liver, leafy greens, broccoli* |

| | |
|---|---|
| Beta carotene | An antioxidant that can be converted by the body to vitamin A as needed<br>*Source: leafy vegetables* |
| Biotin | Metabolizes amino acids; needed for normal hair production and growth<br>*Source: egg yolk, liver* |
| Choline | Prevents fat accumulation in the liver; a major neurotransmitter in the brain<br>*Source: egg yolk* |
| Folic acid | Necessary for proper red blood cell formation; plays a role in the metabolism of fats, amino acids, DNA, and RNA; needed for proper cell division and protein synthesis<br>*Source: grains, peas, beans* |

**TABLE 3.3** *Minerals We Need for Good Health*

| | |
|---|---|
| Calcium | Builds strong bones and teeth; aids in muscle contraction and nerve transmission<br>*Source: milk, yogurt* |
| Chromium | Interacts with insulin to regulate blood sugar levels<br>*Source: nuts, mushrooms, raisins* |
| Copper | Involved in multiple enzyme systems<br>*Source: organs, cereals, nuts* |
| Iodine | Needed for proper functioning of the thyroid gland and production of thyroid hormones<br>*Source: kelp, iodized salt* |
| Iron | Prevents anemia; needed for the transport of oxygen throughout the body<br>*Source: red meat, liver* |
| Magnesium | Needed in many enzyme systems; essential for heartbeat and nerve transmission<br>*Source: nuts, seeds, leafy greens* |

*(continued on next page)*

**TABLE 3.3** *Minerals We Need for Good Health (continued)*

| | |
|---|---|
| Manganese | One factor in the enzyme systems that impact bone formation, produce energy, and metabolize protein<br>*Source: nuts, ginger, tea* |
| Phosphorus | Maintains strong bones and teeth; necessary for muscle and nerve function<br>*Source: meat, dairy* |
| Potassium | An electrolyte needed to maintain heartbeat, fluid balance, and nerve transmission<br>*Source: bananas, orange juice, potato* |
| Selenium | An antioxidant that protects vitamin E<br>*Source: fish, red meat, poultry, Brazil nuts* |
| Zinc | An insulin component that's required for blood sugar control<br>*Source: oysters, beef, turkey* |

Eating nutritious foods loaded with antioxidants, vitamins, and minerals will help you remain vigorous, enthusiastic, and full of joy, even into a *very old age!*

4

# Move That Body

*The Best Prescription for Healthy Aging*

Dear Ageless:

I used to be a ball of fire, but the older I get, the more sedentary I've become. I'm only 65, but I'm tired and not interested in doing anything but watching TV. What's happening to me?

An Unhappy Couch Potato

Dear Unhappy Couch Potato:

An inactive lifestyle becomes habitual, and this can adversely affect physical health in four areas: strength, balance, flexibility, and endurance. Being sedentary also puts you at risk for a variety of diseases and disabilities. Exercise is the best prescription for maintaining good health. It improves lung, heart, and vascular function; increases muscle strength and bone density; and keeps the body limber. People who exercise often look younger, have more energy, sleep better, and have fewer medical issues. They also have a positive attitude because exercise produces endorphins that relieve depression.

Begin with a complete physical exam so that other causes of your lethargy can be ruled out. Discuss exercise with your doctor, who can recommend a personal trainer or fitness coach. Even small changes in your level of activity can be beneficial, such as adding regular gardening, heavier housework, or chasing grandkids. Start slowly, but build to 30-40 minutes at least three times a week. The latest research suggests that fitness can be attained by walking briskly for 30 minutes five times a week.

*Ageless*

*Tai chi is a series of postures or movements (and there are over 100 of them from which to choose) performed in a slow, graceful manner. Each posture or movement flows into the next without pausing. Tai chi doesn't take great physical strength or coordination. Tai chi can reduce stress and increase a feeling of well-being, improve muscle strength and definition, and increase flexibility, energy, stamina, and agility.*

Aerobic activity—such as walking (with a goal of 10,000 steps or 5 miles daily), swimming, cycling, and dancing—improves overall health and builds stamina, allowing us to handle daily tasks and maintain our independence as we grow older.

Weight training builds lean body mass, increases strength and promotes self-reliance, and it jump-starts your metabolism, which will help keep your weight and blood sugar in check.

Yoga and Tai chi are effective for balance and staying flexible, which can help you avoid falls and injuries. These forms of mild, movement exercise are especially useful for seniors because they are so gentle.

Tai chi is a series of postures or movements (and there are over 100 of them from which to choose) performed in a slow, graceful manner. Each posture or movement flows into the next without pausing. Tai chi doesn't take great physical strength or coordination. Tai chi can reduce stress and increase a feeling of well-being, improve muscle strength and definition, and increase flexibility, energy, stamina, and agility.

Some forms of Tai chi are faster than others, although most forms are suitable for everyone. All the forms include rhythmic patterns of movement, which are coordinated with breathing.

Exercise is vital in slowing down and even reversing the impact of the aging process. Greater physical strength is the best medicine for protecting health, staying independent, and keeping your zest for life.

There is no truer cliché than "move it or lose it." Much like the Tin Man in *The Wizard of Oz*, the more sedentary we are, the more immobile our bodies become.

The exciting news is that it doesn't take much effort to recapture some of what you might have lost. The key is to choose physical activities that you will enjoy over the long term. If you exercise just because you think you "should," rather than because you want to, you probably won't do it consistently, and consistency is the secret to any successful exercise program. It's better to walk fast for 30 minutes every day than to spend 3 hours in the gym, be sore and uncomfortable for several days, and not go back.

## BREATHING TO LIVE

Before discussing how to exercise properly, we need to consider an even more basic problem. As we grow older, we begin to do the one thing wrong that harms our skeleton, internal organs, attitude, energy, and sleep patterns the most. We stop breathing—or, more correctly, we stop breathing *deeply*.

As youngsters, our energy level, livelier step, and more physical activities required that we breathe deeply. As we age, we exercise less and take in less oxygen as a result. If our posture also becomes stooped, our ability to breathe deeply is diminished even more because we've constricted the space in which our lungs can expand.

Because breathing is primarily an involuntary activity, we often take it for granted. This is a terrible mistake. Most of us use only 10 percent or so of our total lung capacity, which upsets the ideal balance of gases in the bloodstream by preventing the removal of harmful substances. Taking in more oxygen helps cleanse the body of a variety of waste products, including carbon dioxide.

Storing toxic substances that should be eliminated from the body can diminish mental clarity, lower vitality, and increase anxiety. In addition, fast, shallow breathing can cause sleep disorders and exhaustion, stomach upset and gas, muscle cramps, chest pain, dizziness, and increased heart rate and blood pressure. Some people who think they might have heart disease may actually be experiencing the effects of breathing improperly.

The most important advantage of breathing deeply is that it improves the overall function of your *cardiopulmonary* system (heart and lungs). When we take in oxygen, it enters millions of tiny air sacs (called *alveoli*) and the blood vessels that surround them within the lungs. From there, it passes first to the heart and then throughout the body to the muscles, organs, nerves, and brain.

Shallow, or "chest" breathing, doesn't allow oxygen to reach the lower part of the lungs and fully saturate the blood with oxygen. As a result, you breathe more rapidly, which can increase blood pressure and pulse rate. Your organs must work much harder to increase the level of oxygen in the blood. Over time, this pattern can damage your lungs and heart, diminish your energy, and increase your stress level.

Your entire system will function with greater ease if you breathe deeply, so that the lower part of your lungs fills with oxygen, Your heart will beat more slowly, and your blood pressure will decrease.

In her book *Serenity to Go: Calming Techniques for Your Hectic Life*, Mina Hamilton, a long-time yoga instructor, describes the physiology and impact of deep breathing:

> Deep or diaphragmatic breathing enhances what is often called the "relaxation response," which is basically the opposite of the "flight or fight response," the reaction that allows an organism to respond to real danger.

This system is functioning properly when, for example, you respond to an out-of-control car veering in your direction by leaping to safety. Your respiratory rate jumps in such a situation, which can cause you to gasp for breath. Your heart rate and blood pressure will increase, and your body will be flooded with adrenaline and other stress hormones. Your pupils dilate so you can see better, and your sweat glands spring into action. You literally get "hot under the collar." This is a highly desirable response in a true emergency such as avoiding an accident.

In the relaxation response, your body responds with almost the exact opposite of the flight or fight response. Your respiratory and heart rate slows, blood pressure dips, pupils contract, and you sweat less. Your body comes out of emergency mode. Slow steady breaths help us to be calmer and more serene—even during a crisis. By encouraging this response, you can begin to reverse the adverse health effects that may have built up over many years.

The good news is that you can initiate this calming response, at will, by changing your breathing pattern. Normally, we breathe without conscious thought. No matter what we're doing—sleeping like a log or dancing up a storm—our lungs take in oxygen and pump out carbon dioxide. This is called an *automatic* function. It's how the heart—with no say-so from us—keeps the blood circulating, the liver making enzymes, and the lungs automatically inhaling and exhaling.

Although breathing is automatic, we can also control our breathing. We can hold our breath as we dive underwater to look at a reef fish, or slow it down to deliver that high note when we are singing. We can also change the quality of our breathing to help us be more serene in the midst of what a moment before was a crisis.

When you fully exercise your lungs by breathing deeply, your entire respiratory system becomes involved, even the parts of the lungs rarely used by most people. Because oxygen is the most vital nutrient for our body, the benefits for inhaling as much and as deeply as possible are numerous:

▶ Increases your energy level immediately, and better than any food or supplements

▶ Boosts overall vitality

▶ Removes toxins effectively and eliminates metabolic by-products from the body

▶ Develops chest muscles and improves posture

▶ Increases lung capacity

▶ May diminish respiratory problems such as colds and bronchitis

▶ Reduces the risk of pneumonia, which can be fatal in the elderly

▶ Enhances circulation, and may lead to improved nervous system function because the brain needs three times more oxygen than other tissues of the body

▶ Aids digestion and absorption of food from the gut

▶ Helps to clear and brighten the complexion, and may decrease wrinkling

▶ Reduces stress and relaxes your body by decreasing blood pressure and heart rate

▶ Increases your ability to manage pain

▶ Helps to improves mental capacity and brain function

▶ Helps to promote metabolism by boosting fat burning and weight loss

▶ Reduces anxiety, stress levels, blood pressure, and the heart's workload

Reducing anxiety is critical for many reasons, but modern life makes this difficult. Many people are stressed most of the time. Difficult jobs, multiple jobs, household responsibilities in addition to working, caring for children in single-parent homes, or having to raise grandchildren are examples of why life is far more complicated and anxiety-provoking than ever before. The chronic anxiety these situations produce drains our energy, damages our bodies, and depletes the hormone *cortisol*, which causes an imbalance in glucose metabolism, resulting in weight gain. See *The Cortisol Connection* by Dr. Shawn Talbott for more suggestions about how to reduce stress in your life.

## Breathing Better

The human respiratory system was designed so that we would breathe through our nose, which acts as a filtering system. The hairs that line our nostrils filter out substances that could injure our lungs, such as dust, dander, dirt, and even germs. In addition, the *septum* (the cartilage wall separating the nostrils) has mucous membranes that warm and humidify the air we breathe before it enters our lungs.

Breathing through the nose also helps maintain the correct balance of oxygen and carbon dioxide in the blood. If we release carbon dioxide too quickly—which happens when we breathe more quickly and in greater-than-normal amounts through the mouth—the blood vessels carrying blood to our cells constrict, and the oxygen it contains does not reach the cells in sufficient quantity.

To ensure that you are able to breathe as deeply as possible, you need to resolve any issues that might interfere with proper breathing:

*Reducing anxiety is critical for many reasons, but modern life makes this difficult. Many people are stressed most of the time. Difficult jobs, multiple jobs, household responsibilities in addition to working, caring for children in single-parent homes, or having to raise grandchildren are examples of why life is far more complicated and anxiety-provoking than ever before. The chronic anxiety these situations produce drains our energy, damages our bodies, and depletes the hormone cortisone, which causes an imbalance in glucose metabolism, resulting in weight gain.*

▸ *Avoid foods that inflame the nasal passages and create phlegm.*

▸ *Use a Neti pot to clear your sinuses and nasal passages.* This is a small, long-spouted kettle filled with lukewarm water that can be used to gently irrigate the nasal passageways. Most pharmacies carry them.

▸ *Cleanse the nose with saline solution* to flush out substances that can cause sinus infections.

▸ *Invest in a humidifier.* Dry or overheated air makes breathing more difficult. Be sure it's easy to keep very clean in order to avoid mold formation.

▸ *Avoid breathing chemicals and pesticides.* For example, if you have your home treated for insects, leave until the chemicals have settled or evaporated.

▸ *Stop smoking*—NOW, and avoid secondhand smoke.

Breathing deeply is not difficult. Even babies can do it correctly. In fact, they automatically breathe through their noses (watch when they have bottles or a pacifier in their mouths), and they breathe so deeply that you can see their abdomens rise and fall. We need to duplicate how a baby breathes. This is called "deep belly" breathing.

For adults, this requires awareness and a little practice, because most of us stopped breathing properly long ago. Begin with the simple procedure described below to experience breathing through your nose, emptying your lungs, and using your stomach.

### Breathing Through Your Nose

1. Take a deep breath. Slowly inhale to a count of 5. Relax your abdomen as you inhale. Fill your lungs with air.
2. Slowly and completely exhale to a count of 5. As you exhale, tighten the muscles in your abdomen. Exhale all the air from your lungs. Squeeze your abdomen in and up, and exhale completely through pursed lips. Squeeze hard!

3. Inhale slowly to a count of 5. Relax your stomach. Let it expand and fall as you inhale in a slow and deep manner. Inhale slowly and deeply, completely filling your lungs with air.

4. Now, exhale slowly and completely to a count of 5. As you exhale, tighten up the muscles in your abdomen. Exhale all of the air out of your lungs. Squeeze! Squeeze out all the air. Exhale completely! Feel the power of the exhale. Feel the emptiness in your lungs.

5. Repeat this breathing cycle 3–6 times. Return to your normal breathing as you sit or walk. Your body will be noticeably more relaxed.

## Breathe Away Stress

We know stress wreaks havoc on the mind and body, but we tend to believe we will no longer experience stress once the "stressor" is out of our lives. This is not true. Stress becomes cyclic and systemic, and the damage will worsen if we don't take steps to correct the changes that occur in the body. This can include the depletion of body nutrients, increased insulin sensitivity (which can lead to diabetes), spikes in cortisol and adrenaline (which result in adrenal fatigue and other conditions if the stress is sustained), insomnia, chronic pain, gastrointestinal tract issues, and depression.

Karen Van Ness, a certified fitness trainer and specialist in performance nutrition with the International Sports Sciences Association (ISSA), believes stress is the main reason that headaches, as well as neck, shoulder, chest, and back pain, are now so prevalent. She doesn't believe stress is the only reason for these maladies, however.

Modern technology keeps many of us sitting for most of the day, and sitting for long periods of time is hard on the back. The foundation of our body and the center of our nervous system—the spine—begins to lose its resiliency. This can result in decreased energy, backaches, headaches, neck and shoulder tightness, and even moodiness, irritability, and the inability to concentrate or focus. Visit Karen's website, www.bestbreathingexercises.com, for more information.

Van Ness developed the following exercises, which she calls deep breathing and dynamic, to increase "lung capacity and power, strengthen the entire torso, and promote the unobstructed flow of internal energy that may have been blocked because of systemic stress."

She also suggests that you "Perform these exercises when you first wake up to get rid of the stale air and mucus that has formed through the night, and to break through the wake-up doldrums and ramp up your energy level."

### Morning Exercise

- ▶ *Step 1:* Lie on your back with your arms and legs extended and relaxed. Begin to inhale and exhale smoothly and deeply to the following count: Inhale for 4, hold for 2, Exhale for 6.
- ▶ *Step 2:* To help make sure you are inhaling and exhaling as deeply and completely as possible, place the palm of one hand on your lower abdomen, about 2 inches below your navel. As you breathe, think of inhaling into this point, and exhaling from this point.
- ▶ *Step 3:* Once you have the basic breathing pattern down, add this visualization:
  - *With the Inhalation:* Imagine clean, white, healing, purifying air entering your lungs and then your entire body. The air is sparkling with energy. With every breath, you pull in more of that energy.
  - *With the Exhalation:* Imagine a black cloud of negative energy, toxins, and impurities is being expelled from your body.

As you continue to breathe, feel and see your body becoming cleaner and more energized as you take in clean air and sparkling energy, and force out impurities, toxins, and negative energy. Your body will become filled with healing blue air—like the relaxing beautiful blue of a clear sky on a perfect day.

At this point, you should feel relaxed but energized. Mentally rehearse your goals or objectives for the day immediately after completing this exercise. See yourself achieving these goals and taking any obstacles in stride.

---

**Breathe Better to Improve Health and Attitude**

▶ *Step 1:* Start with your hands hanging at your sides. Inhale deeply for a count of 4. As you inhale, move your arms out to the sides, palms up. Continue moving your arms over your head until your fingers almost touch. Stretch your arms out wide, and then up very high, so that you really expand the chest and lengthen the spine. When your hands are directly above your head, your palms are should be facing down.

▶ *Step 2:* Exhale to a count of 6. As you exhale, push your palms straight down in front of you. Imagine you are helping to push the air out of your lungs until they are completely emptied. Push your palms down to the level of your abdomen. Then move hands to your sides. Repeat.

▶ *Step 3:* Once you have this basic breathing and movement pattern down, add this visualization:

  – *With the Inhalation:* Imagine clean, white, healing, purifying air entering your lungs and then your entire body. The air is sparkling with energy. With every breath, you pull in more of that energy.

– *With the Exhalation:* Imagine a black cloud of negative
energy, toxins, and impurities being expelled from
your body.

As you continue breathing, visualize your lungs
becoming cleaner and clearer as you take in clear air and
sparkling energy, and force out impurities, toxins, and negative energy. Your lungs are now filled with healing blue air—
like the relaxing beautiful blue of a clear sky on a perfect day.

After your lungs are feeling great, extend the healing
blue color throughout your body. If you find a place that is
particularly tight or painful, breathe the healing energy into it.

This is a great exercise to do on a daily basis. You can use it whenever you need an energy boost and need to de-stress or relieve pain. It
will maximize your energy levels and can be used as a quick "pick me
up" when you feel yourself starting to fade.

One of the most effective ways to strengthen your body is to com-
bine regular deep breathing exercises with an aerobic workout. This will
increase your lung capacity and create power throughout your entire
torso. Adding targeted visualization will make your workout even more
effective.

## Breathe Better to Help Control Your Weight

We don't normally think of breathing deeply as exercise, but it is—and
a most effective one at that when it is part of a weight loss or weight
control program. When we breathe deeply, we expand our lungs and
significantly increase the amount of oxygen that enters the blood and is
transported throughout the body. When oxygen reaches our cells, they
use it to do the work for which they were designed—such as rebuilding
tissue. They get the energy they need to function properly from stored
fat, even during low-demand activities.

It's critical to understand that when you are stressed your body does not generally burn fat. Instead, it burns *glycogen*, a form of glucose that acts as an energy reserve. This reserve can be quickly tapped to meet a sudden need for energy.

Your body burns fat when you are relaxed. That's why yoga, which incorporates deep breathing in all its movements, is effective both for weight reduction and muscle strengthening.

Deep breathing should not replace exercise, but it's an effective adjunct to an exercise program, and a good way to begin a new program. If you are not used to exercising regularly, begin with five deep breaths each morning for a week. Note how you feel. Then add five more breaths for 2 weeks and reassess how you feel. If you're not having difficulty, try the exercises outlined above. After checking with your physician, and becoming stronger, add deep breathing to a 30-minute walking routine. The results will astound you.

*Your body burns fat when you are relaxed. That's why yoga, which incorporates deep breathing in all its movements, is effective both for weight reduction and muscle strengthening.*

## Adding Exercise

Historically, people didn't need to think about adding exercise to their daily schedule. Children were not obese because they walked to school instead of riding in cars or buses, and they played outdoors instead of sitting in front of a television or computer.

Chores at home were not simplified by appliances of every sort. Moms raised their own vegetables and ran after toddlers, instead of dropping them at day care and sitting behind a desk all day. Dads pushed a lawn mower and held jobs that were more physically demanding.

The Information Age immobilized us. We sit in chairs in front of screens (computers, BlackBerries, and telephones) at work all day, and we sit in chairs in front of more screens (television, Internet, and play boxes) to be entertained all night.

For the most part, city dwellers and workers walk throughout the day—from the parking lot to the office, to shop, and to run errands. It's often easier and cheaper to walk a few blocks than wait for a cab or subway. In this way, exercise can be structured into the daily routine.

The problem is more of an issue for people who live in the suburbs. Because they are spread out, it's too far to walk to the office or "run" (once a literal term) to the store. Walking to the bus stop used to provide at least some movement, but now most public transportation is limited, and three- and four-car families are the norm.

Suburbanites drive everywhere, and they like it—for the independence, the comfort, and the convenience. The price we pay is limited physical movement during the day. We drive to work, drive through the fast-food line for dinner, and drive to do our errands. We sit in the car. We sit at our desks. We sit in front of one of our various screens at home. We've stopped moving, and we're paying for it with weight gain, diabetes, and cardiovascular disease.

Because of the changes in how we now conduct our lives, we must create time for physical exercise—a mindful, deliberate plan that forces us to get moving. It doesn't have to be a routine in a gym or a work-out designed for the hardiest body builder. A moderately challenging routine that breaks a sweat and lasts about 30 minutes a day is all we need to maintain good health.

Doing a moderate amount of exercise is not only beneficial for maintaining physical health, but mental health as well. The advantages include:

- ▶ Strengthening the heart and lungs
- ▶ Controlling body weight
- ▶ Lowering blood pressure
- ▶ Reducing the level of blood lipids
- ▶ Achieving better control of diabetes
- ▶ Preventing coronary heart disease and stroke
- ▶ Preventing osteoporosis

- ▶ Reducing the risk of falls
- ▶ Rejuvenating the mind and alleviating stress
- ▶ Improving sleep
- ▶ Increasing energy
- ▶ Enhancing the chance of making friends and creating a social circle

## Guidelines for Exercising

- ▶ *Consult a doctor for medical advice before beginning an exercise program.*
- ▶ *Consider inviting a friend or friends to join you.* It will encourage accountability and be more fun.
- ▶ *Wear properly fitted sportswear and sports shoes.*
- ▶ *Pay attention to your safety.* Remove all obstacles in the exercise area.
- ▶ *Start with simple exercises,* and add more as you feel comfortable.
- ▶ *Warm up and cool down,* to minimize soreness and avoid strain. Add stretching exercises before and after exercise.
- ▶ *Breathe deeply while you exercise,* but beware of feeling dizzy, having shortness of breath, and feeling chest tightness. If you have any of these symptoms, stop exercising immediately and consult your physician.

## Aerobic Exercise

Modern technology has simplified our lives, made doing things easier, and given us more time. You'd think we would have filled that extra time with activities that renew and rejuvenate the mind and body. Examples could include organized sports, spiritual pursuits, and family activities. For most people, this hasn't been the case. People often fill their time with even longer work hours, sometimes a second job, and chauffeuring youngsters from one activity to another in increasingly more complicated schedules. Often, for baby boomers and their children, fitting in an exercise program seems overwhelming, or even impossible, after putting in a long day at work, getting the family fed, and doing household chores.

The answer to this problem may have some basis in research, as reported in the *Journal of Applied Physiology* by Kazushige Goto of the University of Tokyo.

The study compared the workout sessions of seven healthy men with an average age of 25. Their respiratory gases and heart rate were monitored and blood samples taken while they performed the following exercise routines:

▶ A 60-minute workout on a cycling machine, followed by a 60-minute rest period (single)

▶ Two 30-minute workouts on a cycling machine with a 20-minute rest in between, and a 60-minute recovery period at the end (repeated)

▶ A 60-minute rest period (for control purposes)

Participants in the repeated exercise sessions had a greater amount of fat breakdown (or *lipolysis*) than the participants engaging in the single exercise session. The two shorter sessions resulted in a dramatic increase over the single session in the release of fatty acids and glycerol, which happens when stored fat is burned. Also, during the repeated session, levels of epinephrine increased and insulin decreased much more than during the single session—a combination that may have further contributed to fat breakdown.

These findings could change the way we approach exercise. Current recommendations by The American College of Sports Medicine to exercise for 45–60 minutes might not be the most effective approach. Splitting up a longer exercise session with a rest period—this is called *interval training*—may be more successful in controlling and losing weight. Even the hardiest athlete could benefit from combining endurance and interval training.

This is good news for people who do not like to exercise, for those who like it but have trouble fitting it in, and for people who want to get fit but want or need to start slowly.

The optimal goal is to get in 30–40 minutes of aerobic exercise four or five times a week. You can divide that work-out time into three parts. For example, take a brisk 10-minute walk or use your treadmill before your shower in the morning. Walk the halls of the building in which you work, or outside if the weather is nice, for 10 minutes after you eat lunch. This can burn off the calories you consumed during lunch more effectively. Then, do a breathing routine (also considered aerobic) for an additional 5 minutes. Not only will you get your exercise and feel energized for the afternoon, but you will also rev up your metabolism throughout the day and burn far more calories.

This leaves just 10 minutes. After dinner, put on some fast music and dance with your spouse or your children. You will all have a ball while creating fond memories, and you will have gotten in your 40 minutes of exercise with no sweat. (Well, actually, you do want to work hard enough during each 10-minute exercise period to break a sweat.)

## Don't Resist Weight Training

Resistance training builds muscle. The more muscle you have, the greater the number of calories you burn throughout the day. If that's not enough reason to lift weights, researchers have also found that resistance training actually *rejuvenates* muscle tissue in healthy, older people.

Dr. Simon Melov of The Buck Institute and Dr. Mark Tarnopolsky of McMaster University Medical Center recently conducted a study to examine the genetic profile of disease-free, older individuals. They took tissue samples from 25 healthy men and women (older than 65, with an average age of 70) before and after 6 months of twice-weekly resistance training, and compared them to tissue samples taken from younger, healthy men and women (20–35, with an average age of 26).

At the start of the study, the older adults showed a significant decline in the function of the components of cells (the *mitochondria*) when compared with the younger people. After the exercise program, however, there was an improvement in tissue function and a remarkable reversal of the genetic fingerprint back to levels similar to those seen in the younger adults.

The surprised researchers had expected the genetic fingerprint to stay fairly steady in the older adults. The fact that they reversed so dramatically gives credence to the value of exercise not only as a means of improving health, but also of reversing the aging process itself.

## Exercises to "Rev Up" Your Metabolism

After age 40, our metabolism slows down at the rate of 2–5 percent *per decade*, and that's assuming your life has not been further complicated by other medical issues, such as thyroid disease, which can also affect your metabolic rate.

Engaging in aerobic exercise 4–5 days a week burns the calories you consume during the week, so that you will maintain or decrease your weight. It increases metabolism during the workout itself, and afterwards as well.

Lifting weights or doing other strengthening activities on a regular basis will boost your *resting metabolism*, which is your basic rate of metabolism when you aren't doing anything at all. This occurs because these activities build muscle, and—pound for pound—muscle burns more calories than fat, even when you are sitting still. This is why men have an easier time losing weight. They have more muscle at the start of a program than women.

Restricting calories too much will actually slow your metabolism, so rev up your metabolism by eating enough food (at least 1,000 calories a day). Because the body creates a *thermic* effect (the increase in metabolic rate to digest food) after eating, you should eat every 4–5 hours to take full advantage of this process. Eat protein with every meal to build and maintain muscle and create a more active metabolism.

## Integrating Exercise into Your Daily Routine

Weight gain is just one problem that comes from sitting at a desk all day. Dr. Angela Smith, former president of the American College of Sports Medicine, says that "Obese people who work long hours at a desk are not the only ones at risk. There are also lots of skinny people who, because they don't exercise for strength and balance, are osteoporotic fractures waiting to happen."

One modern phenomenon is the deluge of complaints about pain resulting from the work we do each day, including ergonomic issues that adversely affect our bodies. This shows up as tennis elbow, carpal tunnel syndrome, headache, muscle strain, and stiffness.

Dr. Smith suggests the following simple stretching exercises to relieve tension, ward off pain, and boost energy and alertness. Be sure to set your computer or cell phone alarm to go off every hour as a reminder to do them.

### Ergonomic Relief Exercises at the Office

▶ *Stand up and sit down—without using your hands.* This can be a challenge, but if you do it while you're on the phone, no one will know.

▶ *Shrug to release the neck and shoulders.* Inhale deeply and shrug your shoulders, lifting them high up to your ears. Hold. Release and drop. Repeat three times.

▶ *Loosen your hands with air circles.* Clench both fists, stretching both hands out in front of you. Make circles in the air, first in one direction, to the count of 10. Then reverse the circles. Shake out your hands.

▶ *Don't forget your fingers.* Stretch your left hand out in front of you, pointing fingers toward the floor. Use your right hand to increase the stretch, pushing your fingers down and toward the body. Be gentle. Do the same with the other hand. Now stretch your left hand out straight in front of you, with your wrist bent and fingers pointing skyward. Use your right hand to increase the stretch, pulling the fingers back toward your body. Do the same on the other side.

▶ *Release the upper body with a torso twist.* Inhale and, as you exhale, turn to the right and grab the back of your chair with your right hand, and grab the arm of the chair with your left. With eyes level, use your grasp on the chair to help twist your torso around as far to the back of the room as possible. Hold the twist and let your eyes continue the stretch. How far around the room can you see? Slowly come back to facing forward. Repeat on the other side.

▶ *Do leg extensions—work your abs and legs.* Grab the seat of your chair to brace yourself and extend your legs straight out in front of you so they are parallel to the floor. Flex and point your toes five times. Release. Repeat.

▶ *Stretch your back with a big hug.* Hug your body, placing your right hand on your left shoulder and your left hand on your right shoulder. Breathe in and out, releasing the area between your shoulder blades.

▶ *Cross your arms—for the shoulders and upper back.* Extend one arm out straight in front of you. With the other hand, grab the elbow of the outstretched arm and pull it across your chest, stretching your shoulder and upper back muscles. Hold. Release. Stretch out the other arm in front of you. Repeat.

▶ *Stretch your back and shoulders with a leg hug.* Sit on the edge of your chair (if it has wheels, wedge the chair against the desk or wall to make sure it does not roll). Put your feet together, flat on the floor. Lean over, chest to knees, letting your arms dangle loosely to the floor. Release your neck. Now bring your hands behind your legs, right hand grasping left wrist, forearm (or elbow if you can reach that far), left hand grasping the right. Feel the stretch in your back, shoulders and neck. Hold. Release your hands to the floor again. Repeat three times or as often as it feels good.

▶ *Look up to release your upper body.* Sit up tall in your chair, or stand up. Stretch your arms overhead and interlock your fingers. Turn the palms to the ceiling as you lift your chin up, tilt your head back, and gaze up at the ceiling, too. Inhale, exhale, release.

## Home Exercises for Adults and Seniors

The Council on Aging and Adult Development of the American Association for Active Lifestyles and Fitness says that functional fitness includes:

▶ Flexibility
▶ Agility and dynamic balance
▶ Coordination
▶ Strength and muscle endurance
▶ Endurance

The Council's Progressive Resistance Training (www.guideline.gov/summary) intervention program describes activities that should begin on a 2-month, three workouts per week basis. During each session, you should complete the following:

▶ *Warm-up.* Five minutes of light exercises designed to prepare the participant for muscle conditioning and to improve overall flexibility

▶ *Muscular conditioning.* Thirty minutes of exercises designed to improve muscular strength and endurance. Most of the exercises use light weights, such as hand-held dumbbells with typical resistance of 1–10 pounds. These exercises are progressive in nature, meaning the participant advances to higher demand levels at their own pace, according to their ability to tolerate the exercises and accommodate the increases in demand. Generally, these exercises are performed for three sets of 8–10 repetitions each, progressing to three sets of 15 repetitions each.

▶ *Cool-down.* Five minutes of light exercises, using some of the same flexibility exercises employed in the warm-up phase. The purpose of the cool down is to return breathing to normal and stretch the muscles worked in the exercise session.

The National Institutes of Health (NIH) recommends four main types of exercise that older adults and seniors can do to stay healthy and independent:

1. *Strength exercises* build muscle and increase metabolism, which helps to keep weight and blood sugar in check.
2. *Balance exercises* build leg muscles, which helps to prevent falls.
3. *Stretching exercises* increase flexibility, alleviate pain, and provide more freedom of movement, which allows for greater activity during our later years.
4. *Endurance exercises* build stamina—walking, jogging, swimming, biking, even raking leaves—any activity that increases heart rate and breathing for an extended period of time. Build endurance gradually, starting with as little as 5 minutes of endurance activities at a time.

### Strength Exercise

▶ *Do strength exercises for all your major muscle groups at least twice a week*, but vary the exercises, so that you don't work the same muscle group 2 days in a row.

▶ *Lift a minimum of weight the first week, then gradually build up the weight.* Depending on your level of fitness, you can start with no weights. Starting with weights that are too heavy can cause injuries.

▶ *Gradually add a challenging amount of weight,* in order to benefit from strength exercises. If you don't challenge your muscles, you won't get stronger. You can build up to using 1- or 2-pound weights as your strength grows and your body adapts to these exercises.

▶ *Take 3 seconds to lift or push a weight into place.* Hold the position for 1 second, and take another 3 seconds to lower the weight. Don't let the weight drop—lowering it slowly is very important.

▶ *It should feel somewhat hard for you to lift or push the weight.* It should not feel very, very hard. If you can't lift or push a weight eight times in a row, it's too heavy for you, and you should reduce the amount of weight. If you can lift a weight more than 15 times in a row, it's too light for you. Increase the amount of weight.

▶ *Do 8–15 repetitions in a row.* Wait a minute, and then do another set of 8–15 repetitions in a row of the same exercise.

## Balance Exercise

▶ Stand straight; hold onto a table or chair for balance.
▶ Slowly bend one knee toward chest, without bending waist or hips.
▶ Hold position for 1 second.
▶ Slowly lower leg all the way down. Pause.
▶ Repeat with other leg.
▶ Alternate legs until you have done 8–15 repetitions with each leg.

▶ Rest; then do another set of 8–15 alternating repetitions. Add weights as you progress.

**Stretching Exercise**

▶ Hold one end of a towel in your right hand.

▶ Raise and bend right arm to drape towel down back. Keep your right arm in this position and continue holding onto the towel.

▶ Reach behind your lower back and grasp the bottom end of towel with your left hand.

▶ Climb your left hand progressively higher up towel, which also pulls your right arm down. Continue until your hands touch, or as close as you can comfortably go.

▶ Reverse positions.

▶ Repeat 3–5 times each session. Hold stretch for 10–30 seconds

## GROWING A HEALTHY BODY

According to *Prevention Magazine*, if you do more in the garden than pulling the weeds and smelling the roses, you can burn 30 percent more calories than during an hour of aerobics, and burning calories is not the only physical benefit.

Gardening is an excellent form of recreation and relaxation. The tranquility experienced while working and walking in gardens decreases tension and lowers your heart rate, increases your ability to concentrate, and can prevent or reverse chronic illnesses such as osteoporosis, arthritis, cancer, and heart disease.

Gardening increases strength, endurance, and flexibility, and the exposure to the sun is an excellent source of vitamin D. But, be sure you wear a hat and sun block to avoid excessive exposure that may lead to skin cancer and premature wrinkling.

*Horticultural therapy* is useful in dealing with emotional issues, such as stress and depression, and it is even effective in improving the symptoms of more extreme mental illnesses. Visit the American Horticultural Therapy Association at www.ahta.org for more information. Working in the garden is also a great way to develop relationships. Friends can share in the effort and the far-superior produce, which will be, hopefully, organic and chemical-free. Grandchildren (even teenagers) will welcome the chance to visit you and play in the dirt. In the process, they'll learn about plants and vegetables, how to care for living things, and accepting responsibility. Most importantly, they'll never forget the time with you and that their effort resulted in such splendor.

> Horticultural therapy is useful in dealing with emotional issues, such as stress and depression, and it is even effective in improving the symptoms of more extreme mental illnesses.

Gardening can be strenuous, particularly if you have mobility or strength challenges. Check with a physician before beginning, and adapt your planning and tools. Consider gardening in a greenhouse or using raised beds and potted containers. Choose a location that has good access (even to wheelchairs) and is easy to prune, weed, and water. Then dig in.

## Exercise for Life

Including exercise in your daily schedule requires thought and a little planning, but the rewards are bountiful: alleviation of aches and pains, weight reduction, strength, and increased energy. Look, feel, and—most importantly—*be* physically younger. You can regain losses in muscle tone and shape, and you will, in a sense, be turning back the hands of time.

Consider swimming for its low-impact advantages, dancing for uniqueness and fun, yoga for deep breathing and relaxation, heavy housecleaning to burn calories and have a spotless home, and gardening for its variety of movement and time in the sun.

Whichever exercise program you choose, begin with breathing deeply and often, and contract and stretch your muscles periodically throughout the day. Mood-elevating endorphins will course through your body, and you'll sleep like a baby.

Most importantly, you will be able to live longer independently. If you exercise your body, even moderately, you will be stronger, more resilient, more capable, and more self-confident—which is the prescription for being able to take care of yourself, rather than needing others to take care of you.

# Part II

## Get Ready for a Fabulous Retirement

# Hitting the Road

## Seeing the World Without Breaking the Bank

Dear Ageless:

Since launching our kids and recently retiring from our jobs, my husband and I have been looking at ways to travel. We don't want to fly, and I get sea sick. Any other ideas?

Getting Antsy

Dear Getting Antsy:

Hop a bus and see America! You can recline in seats that are bigger and more restful for long trips than you'll find on airplanes; stop along the way for breaks, sightseeing, camaraderie, and fun with your fellow passengers; and gaze out enormous windows that allow you to watch the changing countryside of our great land.

Motor coach tours are extremely popular with seniors, because bus travel is safe, comfortable, and a great way to meet new people. They offer the convenience of car travel without the effort of driving.

Custom tours can be organized from budget to deluxe itineraries and from one-day to extended holiday experiences. They *range from limited to all-inclusive packages, which might include accommodations, meals, entrance/activity fees, taxes/gratuities, and an on-board tour guide. Plus, you won't have to guess at costs along the route because they are paid for in advance.*

*Luggage is handled for you at each stop (bus to room and back to bus), and you will be provided with an agenda each day that includes planned activities and free time to explore independently. Breakfast and dinner are generally included in packages, and they can be tailored for special needs, such as low-calorie or diabetic. Be sure to discuss all your special requests when you book the tour.*

*To locate a dependable tour company in your area, call the National Tour Association (NTA) at 800-682-8886 or visit www.ntaonline.com to search for an NTA operator in your area.*

*Motor coach companies are dedicated to selecting the most scenic route, the best accommodations, the finest dining, and all the "must-see" sights possible. They make the arrangements for a fabulous tour and resolve any concerns. You just sit back and enjoy.*

*Ageless*

Many seniors have spent their lives postponing their own needs and desires in order to fulfill family and work obligations. Two-thirds of their lives may have been dedicated to creating a home and collecting things to fill it, raising and launching children, fine-tuning a business or climbing a corporate ladder, and caring for elderly parents and grandparents.

You've earned a retirement that is abundant with peace and pleasure, but that doesn't necessarily mean taking up residence in a rocking chair on the front porch, unless you want to pass an evening that way. It's as important to spice up life after retirement—which may last 30 years or more—as it is to spice up your food for good health.

Keeping your mind and body active may be the best prescription for staying young. Retirement can and should be your time to see the world, have new experiences, and share the knowledge, skills, and wisdom you've gained from a lifetime of learning.

Even on a fixed income, you can experience new places and activities inexpensively. You can study new topics in college classes, which are often free for seniors, learn different skills, participate in unique activities, take a part-time job doing something entirely new—perhaps something you've always dreamed of doing—and give of yourself to others through unlimited volunteer opportunities. You *can* create a retirement that is full, varied, and exciting.

With the same, or just slightly lower/slower, level of commitment that you once directed toward work, baby boomers and seniors can redirect their energy and focus on fun. Travel is a great way to do so.

As described earlier, taking a bus or train to see the beauty and majesty of our country is relaxing and relatively inexpensive. The pace allows for true appreciation of our beautiful countryside, and the available routes and itineraries can take you anywhere you want to go. You can visit Vermont for maple syrup from a tree tap and see the crimson and gold leaves that blanket the winding roads; travel to New York to experience the power of Niagara Falls; peek over the ledge into the Grand Canyon; sample wine in the Napa Valley; or swim in the emerald water of Florida. With a little ingenuity, you can go anywhere.

You can travel in the fall or spring when kids are in school and families must stay home. There will be less congestion on the roads, and you can take advantage of cheaper prices for transportation and lodging, travel while it's cool, and not have to battle crowds.

Besides taking a bus or train, ground travel can also include a car or RV. If you choose this option, make sure the skills of the person driving are sharp enough for long-distance driving, which is significantly different from driving a few miles to the mall. Consider the following list of facts and recommendations from The National Highway Traffic Safety Administration before loading up the car for a road trip:

▶ Drivers older than 70 are involved in more crashes per mile than any other age group.

▶ Many older drivers react too slowly in emergency situations. They cause 14 percent of all traffic fatalities and 18 percent of all pedestrian deaths each year. Degenerating vision, poor hearing, and drowsiness caused by medication are common causes.

▶ Aging affects peripheral vision, light sensitivity, and the ability to focus quickly. A 60-year-old driver needs three times as much light to see as a teenager, and will take twice as long to adjust to changes in light. See your ophthalmologist for a thorough eye exam. She will check for cataracts and glaucoma, visual sharpness, and peripheral vision.

▶ Reacting appropriately is impossible if a driver is unable to hear horns, screeching tires, or sirens. Have your hearing tested by an audiologist and, if necessary, consider getting a hearing aid. The newer models available are smaller, more comfortable, and highly sensitive. Try various types before making a purchase.

▶ Nearly 20 percent of seniors drive while taking medication that can make them sleepy. Driving while drowsy is the leading cause of crashes—and as dangerous as drunk driving.

▶ A physician should determine whether the combination of medications that you take is compatible with safe, long-distance driving.

▶ You should also be examined for chronic diseases such as muscle atrophy, osteoporosis, or arthritis because these conditions can affect strength and flexibility.

Even if everything checks out physically, it may be helpful to take a refresher driving course. The American Association of Retired People (AARP) Drive Safety Program is a good choice. If you are suggesting this for your parents rather than for yourself, include yourself in the plan, because this is a sensitive issue, and you might need to tread lightly. Point out to your parents that the minimum age requirement for the class is 50 (so you will not be alone in this effort) and that a passing grade could mean a reduction in the cost of insurance. For more information, visit www.aarp.org/55alive or call 888-227-7669.

## ALL ABOARD: TRAVEL BY TRAIN

Traveling by train is comfortable, romantic, full of adventure, and fast, particularly if you take high-speed trains. With massive windows on the sides and sometimes on the top of the car, you will have a spectacular vantage point for watching the world go by.

Whether you take the Eurostar from England to France or Holland, the Skytrain across China, the Polar Bear Express to experience an onboard Christmas, or the Trans-Siberian across Russia, you will love the ride.

Train travel between cities in the United States is provided by Amtrak, which has routes all over the country and into Canada. You can check all the schedules and fares online at www.amtrak.com or call (800) USA-RAIL. Amtrak also posts a variety of sales and discounts on its website, so always check to see if there is a special fare to your destination before you make your reservation.

To get the best from your journey, decide in advance which countries or states you want to visit and how much time you will have for each destination. You also need to know when the trains will arrive in various places. Some destinations should be seen in daylight, some in starlight, and you don't want to arrive anywhere in the middle of the night. Imagine the difficulty you might have getting help if you needed a cab or a room for the night.

Overnight trains are a great way to save on accommodations, and sleeping at night is possible on a train. If you sleep when your body is actually accustomed to it, you will have the necessary energy to see those fabulous sights during the day.

Auto trains allow you to take your car with you, and most major airports have convenient train connections into the city. Numerous train passes are available, so you can buy to get the best deal and to ensure that you use all your vacation/travel time to the best advantage.

## Europe by Train

Rail Europe gives the following reasons for seniors to travel by train:

▶ *See Europe on widescreen.* With large windows and everything necessary on board, you can simply reserve a seat, sit back, relax, and enjoy Europe's unique scenery while sipping a favorite beverage.

▶ *Travel in comfort.* You won't feel cramped because the seats on European trains are spacious. You will be free to move around the carriage, or you can just sit back and relax. Some trains have seat-back video and entertainment facilities.

▶ *Dine in style.* You can choose to have a meal in the dining car, have a snack, or enjoy a drink in the bar. Many trains also offer food service at your seat. If you want to save money, take your own food on board.

▶ *A helping hand.* Most trains have a wide range of on-board amenities, including telephones, seat reservation services, and toilets. When you need a helping hand, just ask the conductor.

▶ *Do what you want.* Everyone loves the flexibility of rail's unlimited stopovers, choice of routes, and departure times. It gives you the freedom to stay longer, move on, or revisit a place you like.

▶ *Make the most of your budget.* A range of saver passes and special offers are available to suit almost every budget. If you go with friends, you can save even more by traveling as a group.

▶ *Travel overnight.* Try a luxury sleeper or a more affordable couchette on long overnight train journeys. You'll save on a night's accommodation and arrive at your destination refreshed and ready for the next day.

▶ *Scenic trains.* To truly experience the beauty of Europe, ask your travel agent about special train journeys with spectacular scenery in picturesque countries such as Switzerland and Norway.

▶ *Convenience . . . you can travel all year round.* On the train, you can forget about the hassle of traffic jams or weather delays. Trains operate no matter when you visit Europe, 365 days of the year, come rain, hail, or snow.

▶ *Arrive in the heart of the city.* Most stations are located in the heart of Europe's cities, and they offer a range of services, including restaurants, gift shops, foreign exchange, telephones, post office, bookstores, seating reservations, and general tourist information kiosks.

## Train Travel Tips

▶ *Pick up a copy of USA by Rail* for more information and tips to make your journey a pleasant one.

▶ *Read your ticket carefully* for information regarding reservations, restrictions, amenities, perks, and services.

▶ *Double-check train times and special offers in person when you get to the station.* Schedules and fares may change.

▶ *Ask if reservations are necessary.* A train ticket or rail pass doesn't necessarily ensure getting a seat. Reservations are necessary on some trains, even if the train is not full. If so, make them.

▶ *Anticipate cancellations and delays.* Consider what you will do if this happens. Create a plan and stay cool. Schedule changes are inevitable.

▶ *Plan for enough time between connections.* You don't want to miss the next train.

▶ *Request seating choices.* Remember that seats in most coaches face both backwards and forwards. You can request a window seat or one on the aisle for greater legroom, or you can select two seats separated by a stationary table. First class seats are roomier and generally recline.

▶ *Reserve a sleeper car if you are traveling overnight* and need to be well-rested the next day. Make your reservations well in advance.

▶ *Wear an eye mask and ear plugs to help you get a good night's sleep.*

▶ *Dress comfortably.* It can get cold on a train, so have a sweatshirt or sweater handy, not packed in a suitcase.

▶ *Wear comfortable clothes and shoes.* You may need to move fast, and carrying luggage and negotiating stairs and escalators can be difficult.

▶ *Be sure you can handle your own luggage.* Sometimes, others help us get our bags on board and then—when it's time for us to handle them ourselves—they are too heavy or bulky.

▶ *Buy luggage that can roll and be stacked and secured.* This is particularly important if you must run to make a connection or carry your luggage up stairs in hotels without elevators. (This is more common than you might think.)

▶ *Plan for mealtimes.* Find out the dining car's hours, and schedule your meals accordingly.

▶ *Don't leave your luggage unguarded on the train or in the station.*

▶ *On night trains, secure baggage to the rack* with a lock such as those used for bicycles.

▶ *Keep your valuables in a concealed money belt* while sleeping on trains.

## CRUISING THE WORLD

Taking a cruise is a luxurious way to experience exotic cultures and explore the world. It's an all-inclusive, hassle-free vacation that you can tailor to your needs. Cruises can be value-priced or deluxe, relaxing (lounging by the pool, reading, lectures, and culinary demonstrations), or thrilling (singles parties, gambling, snorkeling and diving, and shore adventures).

Consider a special interest or theme cruise—Roaring Twenties, Big Band, 50s sock hop, arts and crafts, historical, and sports are just a few examples. Single women traveling alone who love to dance can select a cruise line that offers "social hosts" as an amenity, so that they can meet other retired professionals who can provide company for din-ing, dancing, and excursions.

If you are traveling alone, many cruise lines offer stateroom-share options that are economical and a good way to make a friend. They usu-ally guarantee a match with someone of your same gender and smok-ing preference, similar age, and compatible lifestyle.

Ask for a room in mid-ship. It will have greater stability and be closer to the dining rooms and elevators, which is especially important if walking is a problem. Choosing small to mid-size ships is an option for easier access to events, greater senior clientele, and more social inter-action with others. No matter what size ship you choose, check to see if it can accommodate people who use canes, walkers, or wheelchairs.

Diet regimens aren't a problem. Most cruise lines offer flexible dining schedules and menus (kosher, vegan, low-calorie, low-sodium, and fat-free). Discuss any special needs when you make your reserva-tion, three weeks ahead of departure, and again when you board.

Contact your travel agent or cruise specialist for ship options, ratings, costs, and travel tips. Visit www.mustcruise.com/cruise_info/seniors.html, and call 800-365-1445 to ask about AARP member discounts.

## Cruise Travel Safety Tips

One of the advantages of cruise travel is safety. There is very little crime on board, and lots of help if something goes wrong. However, tourists are often targets for thieves and scam artists. Americans are particularly vul-nerable because they are generally friendly and trusting, even of strangers.

Don't be afraid to travel, but do be aware of your surroundings and well-prepared. Some simple strategies and lots of common sense will keep you safe and having a great time. Tips for safe travel include:

▶ *Make copies of your passport, driver's license, and credit cards before leaving home.* Leave a copy at home and in a safe place on the ship.

If the ship's purser holds your passport to expedite clearing the ship in foreign ports, carry a copy of the passport ashore with you.

▶ *Don't buy expensive luggage.* Some thieves equate it with expensive contents. Be sure it's sturdy, though. Bag handlers are rarely careful, and cheap luggage can break easily under the strain. Also, you don't want the contents spilling out unexpectedly.

▶ *Use tape or an extra band to secure your bags, and buy self-locking plastic tags for loose contents.* You can find these heavy-duty items in travel or home improvement stores, or on the Internet.

▶ *Tie something on your luggage that will make it immediately identifiable.* The last thing you want when you're tired, ready to be home, or traveling on to your next destination is to have your luggage pass you by because it looked just like the rest of the bags.

▶ *Don't list your full home address on the outside of your luggage.* This is a signal to expert thieves that you won't be home, making your house their next target.

▶ *Avoid wearing expensive jewelry.* If you want to wear jewelry, take only pieces you wouldn't mind losing.

▶ *Do not flash money.* It's an invitation to pickpockets.

▶ *Take as little cash as you can.* Using a credit card is safer, and you will have a record of purchases and the opportunity to question charges.

▶ *It is best not to take valuables when you travel.* If you must, don't leave them lying around your cabin. Put your wallet and valuables in the cabin's safe or the purser's safe. Remember, in all likelihood you will not be seeing your fellow travelers again. The only people you'll be impressing are the thieves.

▶ *Common sense is needed, even at sea.* Although criminals can't get far, they have lots of places to hide out. Stay in the public areas, and remember that a cruise ship is like a small, unfamiliar city. Its crew and passengers are strangers, so be wary.

▶ *If you are cruising with your children, set rules just like at home.* Meet any new friends your teenagers make and get their names; warn your kids to not accompany crew members to non-public areas; and enforce curfews. Don't give your children "the run of the ship" while you are in the club, show, or casino.

▶ *Do not close your cabin door until you have checked the bathroom and closet for intruders.* Locks on cruise ship cabins are not changed as often as hotel locks.

▶ *Be sure to lock all the doors to your cabin when you are asleep,* including the terrace door if you have one.

▶ *Ask who is there before opening your door.* It's perfectly acceptable to refuse to open the door to someone you don't know. Protect your cabin key and cabin number.

▶ *Be careful in ports-of-call.* Shopping bags and purses are prime targets for cut-and-run thieves, who wait for overwhelmed and distracted tourists in port cities. They will disappear into the crowds with your valuables before you even know you've been robbed.

▶ *Put valuables in a waist pack that locks or threads through your belt loops.* If you carry a handbag, be sure the shoulder strap crosses your body and the purse hangs down the front. Thieves will not have easy access that way.

▶ *Cradle shopping bags in your arms instead of letting them hang from your hands.* Consolidate your bags and walk purposefully, even when you're sightseeing. If you look like a victim, you might become one. Remember, however, if there's a choice between a bag and your safety, let them have it. "Things" are not worth risking your life.

▶ *Men should carry wallets in their front pockets and divide their money between pockets.* It's preferable to carry a wallet that attaches to your belt and tucks inside your slacks.

▶ *Never leave your camera or tote bag on a chair in a restaurant.* Keep it on your lap. If you can't put your camera inside your clothing while walking around, put it in a bag that you wear in the front or in a waist pack with straps that weave through your belt loops.

Although onboard security varies a little from ship to ship, there are cameras that security personnel, officers, and staff can and do visually monitor. They are generally located in the embarkation areas, corridors, public rooms, common decks, pools, and "out-of-bounds" areas for the crew.

There is also strict control of access to ports-of-call and terminals. Passengers are required to show their ID, travel papers if applicable, and tickets to enter both the port area and the terminal, and there are multiple security checkpoints before you are allowed to board the ship.

Embarkation and debarkation may take longer because of additional security procedures. Plan your trip accordingly, and be patient in long lines. These precautions are for your safety, so keep your sense of humor and remember that everyone is—literally—in the same boat!

## Taking Flight

Flying is a common mode of transportation, and sometimes it's the only way to get to the bus, train, or cruise ship that you're planning to take. If you can afford it, or have accumulated enough frequent flyer miles for upgrades, choose to fly business or first class for long flights. Larger seats that recline make sleeping easier, and there is far less noise, commotion, and interruption. If you must fly coach, there are some important tips to follow, particularly where your physical and emotional health is concerned.

*Check with your physician about what medications to take prior, during, and after a flight. Be especially careful about which sleep medications to take, so you don't make jet lag any worse than it needs to be.*

Check with your physician about what medications to take prior, during, and after a flight. Be especially careful about which sleep medications to take, so you don't make jet lag any worse than it needs to be.

## Jet Lag

The symptoms of jet lag include sleep disruption or feeling tired, but there are other symptoms as well—irritability, headaches, difficulty functioning, muscle soreness, and even stomach upset.

Jet lag has no real cures, but there is some agreement about how to manage it:

- *Arrive early to allow time to get adjusted,* especially if you need to be fresh and alert for a business meeting. Be sure to be well rested before you leave home.
- *Drink lots of water*—before, during, and after your flight. Dehydration contributes to the problem.
- *Set your watch to the time at each stop of your journey.*
- *Use headphones, earplugs, and eye masks to block out light and noise.* Try to sleep on the plane at the same time that it would be nighttime at your destination.
- *Eat high-protein foods to stay alert and carbohydrates when you want to sleep.* Try to eat meals close to the time you'll be eating at your destination.
- *Adjust your sleep schedule.* If you're traveling east, try going to bed one hour earlier each night for a few days before your departure. Go to bed one hour later for several nights if you're flying west.
- *Boost your B vitamins.* An over-the-counter vitamin B supplement might help alleviate jet lag.

## Blood Clots

Blood clots most commonly develop in the legs. They are considered an economy-class syndrome because of restricted legroom, and they are more common on long flights. To prevent this potential problem, drink lots of water and move frequently. Stand up and walk around the plane as often as you can.

People with cardiovascular disease are probably already on a regimen of Coumadin® or warfarin, or they are taking aspirin to reduce the potential for blood clot formation. If not, you might check with your physician about taking a "baby" aspirin daily, beginning the week before departure and until you return.

*Ask your physician for a prescription for steroids and antibiotics, in case you have an allergic reaction or become ill with an infection during your trip.*

Any mode of travel can pose emotional and physical challenges. Ask your physician for a prescription for steroids and antibiotics, in case you have an allergic reaction or become ill with an infection during your trip. This is critical, because finding a physician to prescribe medication or a drug store to fill a prescription is sometimes a challenge, depending on your destination. Keep prescriptions in their original containers, so that no question arises about the contents.

## Motion Sickness

▶ Dramamine® (dimenhydrinate) and Bonine® (meclizine) are motion sickness medications that also double as sleep aids.

▶ Transderm Scop® (scopolamine) is a small circular patch you stick behind your ear to reduce nerve activity in the inner ear.

▶ Sea-Bands™ stimulate wrist acupressure points, which are believed to control motion sickness.

▶ Garlic aids in controlling motion sickness and also thins the blood, which is important for those concerned about blood clots; 250–500 milligrams every six hours is suggested. Do *NOT* take garlic if you are taking Coumadin® or warfarin, because it can decrease clotting time to a dangerous level.

## Inability to Sleep

Whether you are trying to rest at an unusual time, minimize jet lag, or avoid listening to the people next to you, sleep aids may be helpful—even necessary—for a more pleasant trip.

The following drugs are effective, but they do have some side effects. Try various alternatives at home to see which works best for you.

▶ Ambien® or Sonata® work well and—unlike Valium®, Xanax®, or Dramamine®—they won't leave you feeling groggy.
▶ Antihistamines such as Sominex®, Nytol®, and Benadryl® all cause drowsiness.
▶ Consider melatonin supplements. The latest research seems to show that melatonin aids sleep during times when you wouldn't normally be resting. Check with your physician about the appropriate dosage, and take it about 30 minutes before you want to sleep.

## TRAVELING WITH DISABILITIES

Travel by people with disabilities is on the rise, and the travel industry is trying to respond with better services and more appropriate accommodations. This is a difficult task, because each person's challenges are different. Therefore, you must be very accurate in describing your individual limitations, because some companies arrange itineraries based on the nature and severity of disabilities.

Contact a travel agent who specializes in working with physically impaired travelers. Visit the American Society of Travel Agents website at www.asta.org and click on the agent search feature.

Although the Americans with Disabilities Act guarantees that disabled travelers have the right to receive equal treatment under the law, the reality is that these travelers still face problems. They might have to deal with difficult or impossible access, inadequate facilities, and possibly higher prices. Some people in the service industry think of people who have a disability with prejudice and impatience.

You *can* take steps to ensure an easier, safer, and more enjoyable trip. Be sure to make your arrangements as far in advance as possible. Discuss your needs at the time of reservation, and call the provider again a few days ahead to confirm that the arrangements are indeed in place. Also, consider purchasing travel insurance in case the trip must be delayed or cancelled.

Be sure to arrive early when traveling by train or air, and be aware of your rights under The Air Carrier Access Act. Note that the Act requires that you give the airline at least 48 hours notice if you are traveling with a group of ten or more disabled passengers. Visit www.dotcr.ost.dot.gov/asp/airacc.asp to download the guidelines to the Act.

Paralyzed Veterans of America provides easy-to-carry cards with the most important points noted. Be aware of your rights, and insist that they be honored. Visit www.pva.org for more information.

## Air Travel

Try to book a direct flight when you travel. Request a seat on the aisle, so that you can get in and out of your seat with ease. If you are unable to walk long distances, prearrange a courtesy wheelchair to be available at curbside when you arrive.

Carrying luggage can be exhausting, so take a minimum of carry-on bags and keep your checked luggage minimal. Some people use a shipping service to send their luggage in advance. Airline regulations are constantly changing, so check with your airline regarding carry-on and checked luggage. Note that extra fees might apply.

Purchase a small, rolling bag to take on board. Stock it with water and favorite snacks. Note that any water purchased outside of the immediate boarding area will not be allowed on board because of safety regulations. The same holds true for any liquid or gel, so check with your airline regarding these rules *before* going to the airport.

Pack prescriptions in their original containers, and bring an extra set of glasses and a change of clothes. Make two photocopies of your ticket, insurance, and credit cards (front and back), emergency contact information, and itinerary. Carry one copy with you, and keep a copy in your luggage. Keep your ticket, boarding pass, and passport in a pouch that can be hung around your neck. Put it under your top layer of clothing, so that it will be protected but easy to get to. Pouches for travel documents are also available in a style that can be worn around your waist under your slacks.

## General Tips

Ask your doctor about ways to cope with any challenges you might encounter, including limited or nonexistent medical facilities in the country you will be visiting, where to get prescription drugs, and potential problems resulting from taking long trips on airplanes and buses.

Check with your insurance company, and with the embassies in the countries to which you are traveling, for names and contact numbers of physicians, specialists, and pharmacies that you might need. Visit Medications for Travel at www.independenttraveler.com/resources/article.cfm?AID=290&category=5m and the Health Care Abroad website at www.cdc.gov/travel/yellowBookCh2-HealthCare Abroad.aspx for more information.

Bring extra medication with you and copies of your written prescriptions as well. Carry them and any medical supplies you need in your carry-on bag. They will be more accessible when carried with you and not in your luggage, in case your checked bag is delayed or lost.

If you're traveling alone, alert the flight attendants about any concerns you might have, and about any help you might need during the flight. Consider carrying a MedicAlert™ card, and wearing a MedicAlert™ bracelet or necklace. They will list your ailments and give a contact number that is answered 24/7 by operators who can answer questions about your health for you if you are unable. Visit www.medicalert.org, or call 800-432-5378, for information about this organization, their services, and available products.

Arrive two hours before your flight time, and check in with the flight attendant when you board and again before you land, for assistance in getting on and off the plane. They can make sure that a wheel-chair is waiting when you arrive at your destination.

Some airlines allow relatives or friends of a special needs flyer to have a one-day security pass that allows them to go to the gate. Be sure to make these arrangements for both departure and arrival. See the resources section in this chapter for three books by Candy Harrington on accessible travel. They provide a wealth of information for people with a range of disabilities.

## INSURE YOUR TRIP

You face two major risks if illness, accident, or emergency strikes during a trip, tour, or cruise—the loss of nonrefundable prepayments for the trip so long planned for, and the heavy expense of emergency transportation to a hospital or back home.

Insurance against these catastrophes comes in two distinctly different forms. *Trip cancellation or interruption* policies are available to cover the losses you would incur if you have to cancel a trip before you leave home, or if you have to cut a trip short.

The other type of coverage comes in the form of *emergency medical evacuation* (EME) policies that pay for the added cost of having to be rushed to a medical facility far from the site of the accident or illness.

## Trip-cancellation Insurance

Trip-cancellation insurance (TCI) reimburses you for whatever your supplier refuses to refund, although you must pursue that possibility first. It pays the difference between what you paid and what you can recover. TCI also makes adjustments for situations such as switching flights or taking alternative transportation, and pays extra costs that might be necessary if your companion has to return home.

TCI also covers you against a wide range of accidents and surprises that might force you to cancel or interrupt a trip: a fire or flood at your house, a call to jury duty, an accident that makes you miss a flight or a sailing, an airplane hijacking, a natural disaster (such as fire, flood, earthquake, or epidemic), terrorism, or a strike.

## Emergency Medical Evacuation

EME insurance is critical to have in case you suffer illness or have an accident during a trip and need onsite help. It will cover the cost of special evacuation, even by helicopter or private medical jet, to the hospital of your choice and your transportation home.

Medical air services companies offer excellent deals, but they are not all alike. Be sure to compare their benefits, exclusions, and costs before selecting one. Make sure also that you are selecting a company that has longevity.

Becoming a member of an association has many benefits. The Medical Air Services Association (MASA) is the first and oldest association of this kind, having been in business since 1974.

When you join MASA, there are no deductibles or co-pays, no claim forms, no age limits, no health questions, and no dollar limits on air transport costs. One low annual fee covers all costs for flights and services, while providing security and peace of mind. All transportation needs are met with the speed of an air ambulance, including vehicle return. Even preexisting medical conditions are covered, beginning 90 days after diagnosis.

Membership in MASA entitles the member to many benefits, and the services are provided by the best-trained personnel. The medical staff is experienced, and they are all Advanced Cardiac Life Support (ACLS) paramedics, registered nurses, and physicians. Trained medical crews, including two medical attendants on every flight, stand by at strategic locations across the nation and around the world, and a team of the most experienced support staff handles medical emergencies every day of the year.

Unlike newer associations that offer emergency air evacuation, MASA also offers non-injury transport for family members, minor children/grandchildren return, escort transportation, ground ambulance (now costing between $600 and $2,000 per ride), mortal remains return, travel expense reimbursement, and worldwide coverage.

Commercial airlines have many restrictions regarding medical patients as passengers, so securing an air ambulance is necessary. The average cost of an air ambulance is $10,000 and could cost as much as $50,000—all paid in advance and covered by few health insurance policies. Depending on the location abroad, the cost of emergency medical care and evacuation could be as much as $175,000. Becoming a member of the association could not only save your life, but also protect you from financial catastrophe. Call MASA at 800-423-3226 for more information.

## TIPS FOR ACHIEVING AN ADULTS-ONLY VACATION

Vacationing with children and grandchildren can be a real treat and an opportunity to make some life-long memories. But there may be times when you want to travel alone or with other adults, and with no kids in sight. Consider the following tips when making your arrangements for an adults-only getaway.

▶ *Do not plan your trip during school holidays* such as Christmas vacation and spring break. Travel can be especially exhausting during the summer, when it is hot and large numbers of families go on vacation.

▶ *September, October, April, and May are the ideal months to travel.* The weather is cooler, kids are in school, and the rates for almost everything drop.

▶ *If possible, travel during the week rather than on weekends.* You'll avoid family travel, and the planes are generally less full.

▶ *The only exception to the rule about traveling during the week applies to visiting museums.* Call ahead to see if school classes are expected to visit, and plan accordingly.

▶ *If you're going to visit a major city, plan your trip for the off-season.* The local people are more patient with tourists, the prices are better, and there are fewer crowds.

▶ *Seek out attractions that are adult-oriented,* such as art galleries, museums, upscale shopping, and clubs.

▶ *Other adult-friendly vacation options* might include a trip to ancient ruins, scientific wonders, a casino, a spa, or deep sea fishing and scuba diving.

▶ *If you want to go to a quiet beach, find more secluded stretches without amusements and snack bars.* Many of the better hotels have private access to the shore and the added bonus of outdoor restaurants and bars on the beach.

▶ *Visit exotic locations.* The longer and more expensive the flight to get there, the less likely families will make the trip.

▶ *This doesn't necessarily mean that you have to go across the globe to enjoy a quiet vacation.* You might consider visiting the less-frequented areas of the destination you are interested in.

▶ *There are still plenty of ships that cater to seniors,* although cruises are becoming an increasingly family-friendly vacation option. Try an upscale luxury line or one that doesn't allow kids under age 14.

▶ *There will be fewer children in restaurants* if you eat later in the evening or pay a little more to eat in nicer restaurants rather than casual chains. Try gourmet or ethnic restaurants.

▶ *When making your arrangements, check the motel/hotel website.* If family packages are offered, you might want to look elsewhere.

▶ *If you can afford it, don't choose well-known budget chains.* Look for intimate bed and breakfasts, historic inns, or upscale hotels.

▶ *When making reservations, ask about the policy regarding children.* This will help you decided if it's the place for you.

▶ *Ask your travel agent about staying at adults-only resorts.*

## Affordable Accommodations

## Bed and Breakfasts

Although an exotic vacation in a far-off place sounds attractive, it's not the only prescription for refreshment and rejuvenation. A change in scenery, attentive service, and someone else in the kitchen can be quite enjoyable, so consider a bed and breakfast (B&B) in a town you've never visited.

The home styles are as varied as the locales. Rustic cabins in the forest, sumptuous villas in the mountains, and charming Victorians with antique lace curtains and embroidered pillows in quaint little towns are just a few of the possibilities

Visit www.bedandbreakfast.com (particularly on Wednesdays, when hot deals are listed) for information about B&Bs in your price and travel range. Then, decide if you'll drive and see the countryside, or fly to another part of the country or world. Be sure to include in your search any special dietary or housing needs, such as disabled access, vegetarian meals, whether or not pets are allowed, and senior discounts.

Ask the innkeeper if the room has comfortable chairs for reading and grab bars in the tub and shower, and whether good lighting is available. This is particularly important in the bathroom to prevent falls during the night. If stairs are a problem, request first-floor accommodations. You may also want to find out if you will have phone and e-mail access.

Although B&Bs can be more expensive than a motel, the ambiance is unique and the meals—if food is served—are often gourmet quality. Rather than choose the least expensive inn or B&B, select the least expensive room in a more expensive one to get the most for your money. The reduced cost in the better inn is generally because you'll have a small room, or you might have to share a bathroom. Typically, even a small room will have a queen-sized bed and private bathroom, and you'll enjoy the same surroundings and amenities as those paying twice the price.

To further reduce the cost, travel off-season and stay mid-week. Ask for a reduction in price for staying multiple nights, and be flexible. Take advantage of last-minute get-away packages.

## Elderhostel

Elderhostel is the world's largest educational travel organization for adults age 55 and older. It's a nonprofit association that has been organizing itineraries for over 25 years, and its expert instructors provide in-depth lectures and lead exciting and often unusual field trips and excursions in over 10,000 programs in more than 90 countries.

The educational programs delve into a wide variety of subjects, including religion, culture, art, food, language, literature, music, and history. Participants are led by university professors, academic specialists, museum professionals, and local scholars. You won't face homework or exams, but the program prides itself on challenging exploration, great camaraderie, and probing discussions that encourage sharing new ideas and experiences.

The types of programs are varied. For example, "Exploring North America" encourages participants to pursue adventure within the United States and Canada. Imagine hiking through the Grand Canyon, seeing the Mississippi from the deck of a paddle boat, or investigating black holes at the Houston Space Center.

You can travel to all corners of the world with Elderhostel's international program—visit Scandinavian palaces, greet Moroccan shamans in Africa, or cross into the Greek Isles to savor Mediterranean cuisine. A cruise ship becomes the classroom in the "Adventures Afloat" program and—if giving service is an interest—programs are available that offer the opportunity to help in struggling communities internationally or within the United States.

Lodging is simple, but comfortable, and might include hotels, inns, and retreat centers, not just dorms on college campuses. Ninety-five percent of the time, participants have private rooms and their own bathrooms. The cut-rate costs for accommodations, three-course meals, gratuities, insurance, lectures, field trips, and cultural excursions are all included.

The value of the Elderhostel programs is extraordinary, given the excellence of the programs and the superior quality of service provided by well-trained staff, who attend to special needs and modify programs for those who are disabled.

Call 877-426-8056 or visit www.elderhostel.org for information about the various programs and to register for your great adventure.

## House-sitting

Being a house sitter is a unique option, not only for traveling the world, but also for immersing yourself in another culture on an extended basis. Property caregivers are in high demand around the world, and seniors are particularly desired because they are considered experienced, trust-worthy, and dependable.

House sitters perform a variety of tasks, including caring for the property, scheduling repairs, protecting possessions, gardening, pet care, and forwarding mail and messages. The sitting duration can vary from one week to a month or more, but—regardless of the length of time—the opportunity to become part of the community rather than just a visitor is invaluable.

Becoming a house sitter is fairly easy. Visit www.housesitworld .com or www.HouseCarers.com for instructions on how to register. For example, with HouseCarers you enter information into your profile (identity and personal information is kept confidential), request desti-nations, and identify the dates you are available. When a prospective homeowner sends a message of interest or a house becomes available, you will be notified by e-mail.

See *The Caretaker Gazette* or visit www.caretaker.org for addi-tional information. Published since 1983, it's the only publication in the world dedicated to the property caretaking field.

## Home Exchange

Another option for affordable housing in far-away places is exchanging homes for a specific period of time. Homes, vacation houses, and even motor homes can be exchanged, and often a car is available for transportation.

Exchanging homes makes dining out unnecessary. You can save hundreds, even thousands, of dollars on hotels, meals, car rentals, and insurance expenses.

Seniors around the country and the world have the same concerns about high-cost vacations. They are even receptive to exchanging hospitality visits for the change in scenery and the opportunity to make new friends.

Visit Senior Home Exchange at www.seniorshomeexchange.com, and see how affordable an exciting holiday can be. This is the only home exchange service exclusively for the over 50-age group.

Wherever you go, and however you get there, travel is one of the greatest experiences you can have during mid-life and as you get older. By taking a few simple precautions before leaving home, any journey can be a safe one. So get going! The world is waiting.

# Pay Back

## *The Amazing Rewards and Opportunities of Volunteering*

Dear *Ageless:*

I'm 63, divorced, and recently retired. I have three children, but they are all grown and live far away. I miss being productive, but don't want the time commitment or pressure of employment. I also miss the companionship I found at work. What can I do to fill the emptiness?

Twiddling My Thumbs and Not Liking It

Dear *Twiddling Your Thumbs:*

Kudos to you for wanting to remain active. It's a critical component of maintaining good mental and physical health. Ensuring that each stage of life is valuable and fulfilling requires making a decision to do something, creating a plan, and then taking action.

Seniors are a precious resource, and sharing work and life experience is a great gift. Seniors have expertise, talent, and time that can be offered to individuals, causes, and organizations that are in desperate need. So consider volunteer work—rocking newborns, reading aloud at the library, or visiting people in nursing homes.

Volunteering reduces depression, increases self-esteem, and improves overall physical health. Seniors who give of themselves to the community are far more optimistic and have a sense of empowerment.

Additionally, often the best medicine for easing the pain of some our own problems is to focus on the needs of others. The opportunity to compare our struggles to those of others gives us perspective and fosters greater appreciation of our own circumstances. Giving to others also adds value to life, redirects self-preoccupation and self-pity, and creates a true sense of satisfaction.

Opportunities to volunteer exist in every interest area and can be local, national, or international. Call Global Volunteers at 800-487-1074 to help change lives around the world, or visit www.greenvol.com to help protect natural resources.

*Ageless*

## BEFORE BECOMING A VOLUNTEER

▶ *Visit the website of the organization you are considering.* It should be professional looking and easy to navigate, and should speak to any concerns and questions you may have. A user-friendly website suggests a legitimate organization, but don't stop there.

▶ *Arrange to visit the agency for which you might volunteer.* Speak with the administrator about the organization's mission and how they view volunteers in the plan to achieve their goals.

▶ *Meet your supervisor.* Discuss what the job entails and how your abilities match, the length of commitment, and deadline requirements.

▶ *Ask if training is available and/or required.* Be clear about the organization's expectations regarding the behavior of volunteers, such as specific requirements regarding interaction with clients, coworkers, and supervisors.

▶ *Even volunteers are interviewed for various positions.* Don't be afraid to discuss your motivation for investing your time and energy. You should be clear about what you are comfortable doing or not doing.

▶ *Although you are going to be working as a volunteer, you are still making an important commitment.* Many volunteer organizations are as big as corporations and as complicated to operate, so people will be depending on you, just as they did in any company for which you might have worked previously. You will be expected to complete your assigned tasks to the best of your ability and meet deadlines.

▶ *If you are still not sure whether the job is right for you, ask about the possibility of trying the position for a while.* Try to make the decision about whether to continue or not as soon as possible. If a trial run is not possible, and you still have misgivings, say no to the position.

▶ *Take your time—not every volunteer job is right for every volunteer.* Be careful and only select a position for which you are capable, particularly in the beginning. You can experiment with more complex assignments after you have had some experience.

Many varied, exciting, and important volunteer opportunities are available—some are even critical to society. The following sections explore just a few possibilities.

## Get Connected

Senior Corps is a national organization that offers three main programs: Foster Grandparents, Senior Companions, and Retired and Senior Volunteer Program (RSVP). According to Senior Corps:

The Foster Grandparent Program connects volunteers, age 60 and over, with troubled or abused children and young people. Volunteers also mentor and help children with exceptional needs, including illnesses and disabilities.

The Senior Companion Program connects volunteers, age 60 and over, with adults in their community who have difficulty with the daily tasks of living. Volunteer Companions make friendly visits, help out with shopping and light household chores, and interact with doctors and pharmacies.

RSVP connects volunteers, age 55 and over, with service opportunities in their communities that match their skills and availability. From building houses to immunizing children and from enhancing the capacity of nonprofit organizations to improving and protecting the environment, RSVP volunteers put their unique talents to work to make a difference.

In addition to making an extraordinary contribution to your community, the benefits of volunteering can include transportation reimbursement, an annual physical, insurance, and—if income-eligible—a modest, tax-free stipend. For more information, call the Senior Corps at 800-424-8867, or visit www.seniorcorps.org or www.joinseniorservice.org.

## OMBUDSMEN IN LONG-TERM CARE

The Ombudsman Program is federally mandated under the auspices of the Department of Aging and Disabilities. It offers an excellent opportunity to advocate for elderly people in long-term care (LTC) situations, such as nursing homes, assisted living centers, and group homes. Ombudsmen advocate for quality care in LTC facilities and for the rights of the residents. They help protect the health, safety, and welfare of LTC residents; resolve residents' complaints; educate consumers; and access state LTC Ombudsman Program resources.

An ombudsman can share vital information about the process for selecting LTC with clients and families, overview the admissions packet, and act as a mediator between the resident and facility staff when problems arise. If problem resolution isn't possible, or the problem involves abuse or complex medical issues, the ombudsman can refer clients and their families to appropriate state agencies.

Because the Ombudsman Program is authorized by federal law, it operates in all states. Call 800-252-2412 for a complete list of residents' rights and to get statewide information throughout the United States.

Volunteers in this program make personal contact with the residents on a weekly basis, so the need for more people to help is huge, particularly because the number of facilities in every state is growing as quickly as the number of older individuals.

## MEALS ON WHEELS

Each day in America, hundreds of thousands of our senior citizens go hungry or are severely malnourished. Vulnerable to disease, disability, and escalating costs, seniors on fixed incomes often have to choose between buying food or medicine. Some are no longer physically able to shop and cook, and others live in remote areas where help is not available.

The Meals on Wheels Association of America (MOWAA) is a nationally networked program dedicated to helping men and women who are elderly, frail, disabled, or housebound. The oldest and largest organization of its kind, MOWAA provides meals and nutritional services, and enhances lives by offering social and economic services.

Under the direction of case managers, an army of caring and cheerful volunteers delivers nutritious meals to the homebound and reports any problems. Just as important, however, they offer the only human contact some of the recipients have.

Eligibility varies greatly, so it's crucial to call your local program. Generally, consideration is given to those who have low-incomes, are in jeopardy of losing their independence, or reside in rural areas. Many programs consider only whether a person is homebound, unable to prepare a nutritious meal, and has no one else to help them.

Dieticians tailor the meals as necessary, including special needs such as diabetic, low-sodium or low-fat, lactose-free, and pureed. Religious/ethnic considerations are taken into account, and additional supplements are available. There are no mandatory costs, and no one is denied service because of inability to pay, but contributions are encouraged.

MOWAA sponsors March for Meals (during March) to raise public awareness about senior nutrition and to collect the funds imperative to feeding so many in need.

For general information, call Eldercare Locator at 800-677-1116, or visit the national organization at www.mowaa.org to arrange services, volunteer, and make donations.

## KEEPING THE FAITH

Faith in Action is a national program that brings together volunteers from different faiths to serve people in need. Sponsored by the Robert Wood Johnson Foundation, the program provides no-cost service to low-income families and the homeless, disabled, and elderly.

The program's mission is to provide emergency services and resolve short-term crises, such as food and financial assistance, and also to educate, mentor, and train people in need. It enables elderly and disabled people to stay in their homes and live independently for longer.

Trained caregivers cannot provide medical help, but they can provide transportation, give respite to family caregivers, run errands and shop, and deliver monthly groceries. They will also assist with paying bills, make supportive phone calls, do minor home repairs, cook, and do light housework in private and group homes or apartments, as well as nursing or hospice facilities.

Volunteers, many of whom are seniors themselves, are extensively screened for the protection of the elderly, and trained by the program directors, who oversee all interactions. According to the organization's guidelines, "When family members and health care providers cannot fill the daily needs of a member of the community, the Faith in Action volunteer fills the gaps. Most belief systems include a mandate to help others. Faith in Action connects neighbors in need with those who want to make a difference."

Faith in Action is based is in Princeton, New Jersey, but the program has spread to all 50 states, plus Puerto Rico and the U.S. Virgin Islands. Visit www.fiavolunteers.org, or call 877-324-8411 for program locations.

## THE AMERICAN RED CROSS "WHEELS" PROGRAM

Wheels is one of many important programs sponsored by the American Red Cross, a volunteer-led organization founded by Clara Barton during the Civil War. Originally conceived to care for soldiers in combat and to aid the victims of war, the American Red Cross is the largest humanitarian aid agency in the world.

The Wheels program provides reliable, door-to-door transportation for anyone who doesn't have access to public transportation and needs to get to a medical appointment. Modified vehicles accommodate elderly and disabled people, including wheelchair users.

Because Wheels is the only countywide service, spaces fill quickly, so people who need services must contact them at least three to five days prior to an appointment to register and set times, and then reconfirm the morning of the day they need the ride. The fare is $2.00–$2.50 each way, but no one is denied access based on ability to pay.

The scope and criteria of programs vary from chapter to chapter, so contact the national office of the American Red Cross at 866-438-

4636, or visit their site at www.redcross.org for valuable information about this program and others, opportunities to volunteer, and how to make a donation.

## Outdoor Volunteering

Many opportunities exist for volunteering in the great outdoors. Whether you work in your own area or in a distant locale, you can hike, backpack, or camp in some of the most beautiful state parks in the nation, and help our country in the process.

The following volunteer possibilities are examples of the thoroughness with which information has been gathered and described by the Lyndon B. Johnson School of Public Affairs at the University of Texas at Austin, and included on the Service Leader website. Visit www.serviceleader.org for some of the best information about volunteer opportunities.

## Volunteers in the U.S. National Forests

Volunteers are the heart of the Forest Service, which matches its mission with your talents, skills, and work preference. You may work on a part- or full-time basis. You can participate in a one-time project or serve over several months, during specific seasons, or year-round. Training may be provided to you if your job requires it. If you are retired or have summers free, you might wish to live in a national forest while you work as a volunteer.

## Wilderness Volunteers

Wilderness Volunteers is an organization that promotes volunteer service in America's wild lands. Volunteers are matched with work projects for public land agencies, such as the U.S. Forest Service, U.S.

Park Service, Bureau of Land Management, and the Department of Fish and Wildlife. The website includes a trip list, ranging from moderate car camping to strenuous backpacking. All trips are led by volunteer leaders in cooperation with land agency representatives. Trips are one week long and are limited to 12 or fewer participants. Participants provide their own camping gear (a list specific to each trip will be mailed with registration confirmation), a sense of adventure, and a willingness to contribute time and energy to worthwhile projects.

## The Council on International Educational Exchange

The Council recruits volunteers from around the world to join projects hosted in various National Forests. Volunteers come prepared to work 30–35 hours a week in exchange for room, board, and the opportunity to learn about the host community.

## Passport in Time

The Passport in Time (PIT) volunteer programs provide opportunities for individuals and families to work with professional archaeologists and historians on historic preservation projects.

## Volunteers for Peace

This nonprofit organization is part of the U.S. Forest Service. It offers over 1,200 short-term voluntary service projects in 70 countries. These International Workcamps are an opportunity to complete meaningful community service while living and interacting in an international environment. Typical work projects with the Forest Service include historic preservation, archeology, and environmental projects such as trail building, environmental education, wildlife surveying, and campground maintenance.

## National Park Service

Volunteers with the National Park Service come from every state and nearly every country in the world to help preserve and protect America's natural and cultural heritage for the enjoyment of present and future generations. Young and old alike give of their time and expertise to assist paid staff in achieving our national mission. This site has a good Volunteering Opportunities section as well as a fine section on Volunteer Management.

## Bureau of Land Management

The United States' federally owned public lands are owned by every American, giving each of us a shared interest in their care and their future. Nearly half of these lands—264 million acres—are managed by the U.S. Department of the Interior's Bureau of Land Management (BLM), making the BLM the manager of the nation's largest land trust. This is a big responsibility.

Fortunately, help is close at hand. Each year, over 20,000 Americans volunteer their time and talent. Working alone or with a group, BLM volunteers enjoy work that matches their interests and schedules. Some volunteers serve part-time, while others enjoy a seasonal or full-time position. The important thing to remember is that even a few hours a month can make a big difference.

## U.S. Geological Survey

The U.S. Geological Survey (USGS) provides the country with reliable scientific information to help describe and understand the Earth; minimize loss of life and property from natural disasters; manage water, biological, energy, and mineral resources; and enhance and protect our quality of life. The USGS's Regional Map can be used to locate volunteering opportunities near you. Submit the application electronically, and a host for each volunteer opportunity you selected will contact you.

## U.S. Fish and Wildlife Service

Volunteers to the U.S. Fish and Wildlife Service develop a greater understanding and appreciation of refuges, hatcheries, and other areas through hands-on experience. Working side-by-side with Service employees, volunteers help protect, conserve, and restore our nation's fish, wildlife, plants, and habitat.

*Visit www. volunteer.gov/gov for a list of volunteer opportunities nationwide.*

Visit www.volunteer.gov/gov for a list of volunteer opportunities nationwide. The mission of this governmental agency is to:

- ▶ Increase the effectiveness of public sector organizations
- ▶ Enhance relationships among different segments of our society
- ▶ Facilitate new approaches for expanding the foundations for volunteer action
- ▶ Broaden the base of the American volunteer movement

You can also contact the regional volunteer coordinator for your state of interest. The Service Volunteer Coordinators are listed at www.volunteer.gov/gov.

## VIRTUAL VOLUNTEERING

If you have a home computer and access to the Internet, the possibilities for volunteering are endless. Virtual volunteering has many advantages, including:

- ▶ *Flexibility*—you can schedule your work when you want or need to.

▶ *Informality*—you could conceivably work in your robe and slippers, because no one will see you.

▶ *Independence*—you will not have anyone hovering over you while you work, and you will not need to interact face-to-face with staff members.

For some people, these differences from the "real" workplace make virtual volunteering ideal. These same reasons can make it difficult for others. Many people enjoy the camaraderie of personal contact, so working exclusively from home might not be particularly gratifying or as much fun.

Additionally, people are often motivated to do their best work by coworkers, the presence of a manager, the fear of losing their job, or the joy of getting a paycheck. None of these motivators exist for the person volunteering from a home office. Being self-motivated is critical, because the organization for which you have volunteered is depending on you just as much as your regular employer once did. You need to be sure that virtual volunteering is really what you'd like to do, so test it out. Take easy jobs at first—short in duration and not too complicated. Then decide.

According to the School of Public Affairs, "Online volunteers can typically be classified as one of two types, depending upon the work they do: technical assistance volunteers and direct contact volunteers," They outline the positions as follows:

▶ *Technical Assistance Volunteers:* These volunteers have a particular expertise and provide assistance with specific assignments. This group may include both on-site and off-site volunteers who can fulfill these various responsibilities:

  – *Conducting online research:* Finding information to use in an agency's upcoming grant proposal or newsletter, gathering information on a particular government program or legislation that could affect an agency's clients, gathering website addresses of similarly focused organizations, and using online phone books and websites to update contact information for a database

– *Providing professional consulting expertise:* Answering an agency's questions regarding human resources, accounting, management or legal issues, writing a speech, developing a strategic plan for a particular department, setting up a video conferencing event, and providing industrial designs

– *Helping with advocacy:* Posting information to appropriate online communities (newsgroups, lists, etc.), preparing legislative alerts to be sent via e-mail, and keeping track of legislation that could affect an agency's clients

– *Translating documents* into another language

– *Providing multimedia expertise,* such as preparing a PowerPoint, Hypercard, QuickTime, or other computer-based presentation

– *Designing an agency's newsletter or brochure,* or copy editing an agency's publication or proposal

– *Proofreading* drafts of paper and online publications

– *Researching and writing* articles for brochures, newsletters, and websites

– *Designing a logo* for an agency or program, or filling other illustration needs

– *Preparing information* for an agency's website

– *Writing a technology plan,* designing a marketing strategy, or directing other types of organizational planning and outreach

– *Making sure a website is accessible* for people with disabilities

– *Registering an agency's home page* and other appropriate pages with online search engines, directories, and "What's New" sites

– *Adding an agency's volunteer opportunities to online databases*

– *Designing a database system* using an agency's in-house database software

– *Providing advanced website programming*

– *Doing regular searches* for news articles relating to an organization or a particular topic

- *Volunteer management assistance:* managing other volunteers in the aforementioned activities, providing an online orientation to all volunteers with Internet access (whether or not they are on-site or online volunteers), surveying volunteers via e-mail about their experiences with an agency or program, keeping track of volunteer hours, and entering volunteer opportunities in online databanks

▶ *Direct Contact Volunteers:* This type of volunteer comes into direct contact with a client or service recipient. For example, via e-mail or a chat room, a volunteer might:

- *Electronically visit* with someone who is homebound, or in a hospital or rest home; this can be done in addition to on-site, in-person visits.

- *Provide online mentoring and instruction* via e-mail or private intranet; for example, help students with homework questions; help an adult learn a skill or find a job; help someone to pre-pare a resume or explore career options; or help prison inmates with studies or programs

- *Help with language instruction;* for example, help someone learn English

- *Staff an e-mail or chat room answer/support line,* such as a phone answer/support line, where people write in questions and trained volunteers answer them; or be part of an online support group, where members provide advice to each other via a chat room, list, or newsgroup

- *Supervise or moderate* an agency-sponsored chat room, e-mail discussion group, or newsgroup

- *Provide advance "welcoming"* via e-mail or a special web page or intranet, for people who are about to enter the hospital or go to summer camp, for example, and also post-service follow-up

- *Work with other volunteers and/or clients to create a project,* such as writing about the news of their neighborhood, school, or special interest group; or gathering history information relating to a particular time or region to post on a website or use in printed material; or train volunteers in a subject via the Internet

## Informal Online Volunteers

Scores of online discussion groups are not formally affiliated with or supervised by any agency. In these groups, anyone can ask questions, and anyone can provide support to others for just about any subject imaginable. These online support groups deal with everything from using a particular type of software, to parents home-schooling their kids, to people with a particular disease, to fans of a particular hobby. People who provide assistance in this type of setting are also volunteers.

To participate, a potential user merely signs up via the web, subscribes via e-mail, or points a newsreader to a newsgroup. From the volunteering point of view, these groups offer many advantages. There is no application or screening process, no set time commitment, and people volunteer whenever and however they like. Numerous people benefit from these informal online groups, which can be of tremendous value to participants.

## Volunteers with Disabilities

People with disabilities volunteer for the same reasons anyone else does. They want to contribute their time and energy to improving the quality of life. They want challenging, rewarding, educational service projects that address the needs of a community and provide outlets for their enthusiasm and talents.

One benefit of virtual volunteering programs is that such programs allow for participation by people who might find other types of volunteering difficult or impossible because of a disability. It also allows organizations to benefit from additional talent and resources of more volunteers.

Harris Poll results from June of 2000 report that 48 percent of people with disabilities who have access to the Internet believe that it has significantly improved their quality of life, compared to 27 percent of adults without disabilities. Therefore, people with disabilities already see the true value of online communication, and they are in a prime position to participate in volunteer projects via the Internet.

The most difficult obstacles to surmount for a person with a disability can be the attitudes of others, such as prejudice and stereotyping. An important part of an organization's efforts to welcome and actively recruit people with disabilities as volunteers is to get a sense of the staff's sensitivity to and knowledge about people with disabilities.

The Youth Volunteer Corps provides two questionnaires to help measure the views of people with disabilities: Scale of Attitudes toward Disabled Persons (SADP), and the Disability Quotient Questionnaire, as well as exercises to encourage staff discussions. These worksheets are available by calling Youth Volunteer Corps at 913-864-4095.

## Tips for Virtual Volunteering

These tips have been compiled by www.serviceleader.org:

▶ *Carefully assess every volunteer project.* It is critical that you consider job expectations and scheduling before agreeing to volunteer for projects—virtual or otherwise. Because you are not working with individuals on-site when completing a virtual project, it is necessary to be task-oriented and highly self-motivated to complete assignments. Even on a virtual project, the organization will rely on you to meet deadlines and complete the project for which you have volunteered.

▶ *Discuss the job description* with your contact at the agency at the time the assignment is made, as well as your expectations and limitations.

▶ *Make sure you understand what your commitment will be.* Don't be afraid to ask questions and seek complete answers. This will cut down on problems you may encounter, or cause for others.

▶ *Expect a period of adjustment.* Even the most motivated and organized person must figure out how to handle a project—the most effective way to manage time and space, orchestrate feedback and communication, and complete project objectives. These logistics are a greater challenge because the work is done remotely, so expect some problems along the way.

▶ *Create a schedule.* When you take on a project, set a specific time frame in which to complete it. Then create a work schedule. When people work at home, it's easy to get distracted, and time does fly. The deadline that seemed so far away at the start might be right around the corner, so consider the following:

   – How many hours will you work on an assignment each day and week? Which hours will you work? How many breaks will you take during your volunteer activity? You can limit your tendency to overwork or motivate yourself to work harder by deciding this up front.

   – Some people are most comfortable with systems and routines that would be very much like those they would use on-site at an agency. You might try counting backwards from project deadlines, and then making careful daily and weekly schedules for what you need to accomplish. Work until you've finished meeting your goals for each day, and then quit.

   – Develop a system for completing and checking your work. Assess it periodically. If something is not working for you, make adjustments. Systems should make your life easier, not more complex.

   – Create mini-goals along the way. Breaking up a massive assignment into manageable pieces increases the probability that you will reach the end goal.

▶ *Do not over-commit.* It's important that you take it slowly at the beginning. Take a short-term assignment—one that will require only a few hours. If you like it, take on something more or a bit more complicated. This will give you a frame of reference for whether this will be work you like.

▶ *Keep a careful record of your work hours.* Then decide how much time you have and are willing to commit.

▶ *Communicate with the organization.* Set up a system for regular contact with the group for which you are volunteering. Be prepared with your questions, and welcome feedback. A positive evaluation will serve as continued motivation.

▶ *Follow the organization's policies.* Every organization has a chain of command and various protocols that must be adhered to, such as how to handle confidential information and how to deal with clients. These policies apply to volunteers in the same way they do to employees. Be clear about what the organization expects from you.

▶ *Avoid burnout.* When you work in an office, there are schedules such as specific starting and stopping times, as well as built-in rest periods. Even on-site volunteers follow prescribed routines. This is not true for virtual volunteers. When volunteering virtually, you may not know when to stop. This can lead to fatigue and burnout, and frustration for the organization if you've committed to a particularly large and important assignment.

▶ *To avoid overwork, set firm starting and stopping times.* Develop a routine and take breaks to avoid headaches, eyestrain, or neck and back pain.

▶ *Motivation from within.* In addition to paychecks and commissions, organizations use various incentives to motivate employees and volunteers. Volunteers who work on-site interact with staff and clients. This creates excitement and inspiration. Volunteers working virtually don't have these natural, informal inspirations, so you will have to be much more self-motivated and self-driven. When you volunteer virtually, you need to be "you own best cheerleader." Tips to increase self-motivation include:

- Begin your task immediately, when your excitement is at its greatest. Reward yourself when you reach each goal.
- If you find yourself having trouble completing an assignment because you just can't seem to get started on it, try re-reading the job description and review the organization's website. Think about what your contribution is going to allow them to do. If you don't know, ask.
- Take breaks to avoid burnout—exercise, make phone calls, play games, visit with family members and children/grandchildren, eat (fruit or protein will help with stamina), drink coffee or tea (caffeine will energize you, but don't take it if it makes you jittery), or take a walk outdoors.
- Give yourself positive reinforcement. Don't berate yourself if you fall behind. Just get back on track.

▶ *Keep your workspace neat and well organized.* Set up your work space so that all your equipment and materials are within reach. Keep things in order, and expect others in your household to respect your work area.

▶ *Decide how and when you will allow interruptions.* Make those decisions clear to your family members. This will model the behavior that volunteer work is serious and important.

▶ *Program evaluation.* If you get a survey from the organization about your volunteer experience or future interests, respond to it candidly. Your feedback will help the organization improve its program. Also, agencies rely on such feedback to help them meet the evaluation requirements for certain grants.

As you grow older, there's no need to resign yourself to boredom or sitting in front of the television all day. The opportunities to give your time and talents back to your community are endless and can be infinitely fulfilling.

# Grandparenting

*The Best of All Possible Worlds*

*Dear Ageless:*

*My three grandchildren, ages 6, 8, and 12, are coming to visit, and I couldn't be more excited. I want to make it an enjoyable time for them, but I also want to make it memorable. What do you suggest we do?*

*A Happy Grandma*

*Dear Happy Grandma:*

*Ideas abound for spending quality time with youngsters. Children of all ages love exploration, and you needn't go far. Rummage in your attic or garage for memorabilia, old clothes, hats, and jewelry to dress up for tea parties or story time about the family. Serve up photo albums and scrapbooks with punch and cookies, and you'll have an event to remember.*

*Explore nearby parks and begin collections. Identifying and displaying rocks, leaves, flowers, or bugs is educational and fascinating for even the youngest scientist. Don't forget a picnic basket filled with snacks and drinks, a kite if it's windy, fishing poles if there's a creek, and a wagon for anyone who might get tired.*

*Investigate your neighborhood library. Apply for library cards—having one makes children feel so grown up—and sign up for story or show time, which are sometimes conducted by costumed storytellers. Check out stacks of books and the library's free videos, DVDs, and cassettes.*

*Search the countryside for working farms that let children milk cows or feed chickens, roadside markets that allow picking fruit or vegetables, and zoos that encourage petting the animals.*

*Hunt through recipes and kitchen-test them. Nothing is more fun than mixing ingredients, punching dough, and eating the product of your efforts. Then "write" a family cookbook. Pepper it with family anecdotes and garnish it with photos of the kids cooking and their drawings of the experience.*

*For more activity suggestions and information about caring for grandchildren, visit www.cyberparent.com. Also read Vicki Lansky's books "101 Ways to Make Your Child Feel Special," "101 Ways to Tell Your Child 'I Love You,'" "101 Ways to be a Special Dad," and "101 Ways to Be a Special Mom."*

*Ageless*

Nothing is more exciting for young children than a visit with grandparents. These are times of pampering and indulgence, novelty and undivided attention, and they are often among the sweetest remembrances of childhood.

The most common focus is on grandmothers, because women (of any age) usually fulfill the primary role of nurturing, teaching, and entertaining children. However, a grandfather can be an important mentor and role model, having a critical influence on his grandchildren's growth and success. According to the American Association of Retired People (AARP), "Grandchildren who have a close relationship with a grandfather are more likely to perform well in school, display positive emotional adjustment, have higher self-esteem, and have a greater ability to develop and maintain friendships."

Grandfathers are often great storytellers. They keep the family's history alive by passing on the details to new generations. They recount firsthand how life has changed culturally and technologically through the ages. They teach powerful lessons by relating the joys, hard times, and even mistakes in their own life experience.

Because grandfathers do not usually have parental responsibilities, their relationships with grandchildren are more open and relaxed. Without fear of judgment and reprisal, grandchildren are more willing to confide fears, ask difficult questions, and entrust their most guarded secrets.

A grandfather's wisdom is highly respected, and his suggestions may be more readily followed. His behavior and actions can set the standard for the kind of man a grandson may become or the kind of man a granddaughter may choose to marry. They have the power and opportunity to teach their grandchildren important life values, such as loyalty, patience, perseverance, and self-sacrifice. Grandfathers should fulfill this sacred obligation to their grandchildren, and their grandchildren should honor them for doing so.

## STAYING IN TOUCH

Maintaining contact is critical if grandparents live too far away for easy visiting. It's important to do it the way the kids do—by phoning, texting, e-mailing, and blogging. If these terms are unfamiliar to you, it's time to get educated and get with it!

Most kids have cell phones, many with texting capability, and some with a feature that allows for retrieving and sending e-mails. Making calls to their cell phones instead of the landline at home allows for a private conversation between you and your grandchild. The reverse is true as well. If the child has something to confide, and you're the adult they trust, they might choose to call you from their cell phone.

Even if grandparents were highly critical of their own children, most treat grandchildren differently. They are more tolerant, more flexible, and more affirming. In fact, most grandparents think their grandchildren are perfect, and this attitude is usually clear to the child. The result is that grandchildren often view their grandparents as their most important confidants, and it's important to foster this trust. Life is tough for kids, and they need people with whom they can communicate, especially if they can't communicate with their parents. The more confidants they have in their lives, the more secure they will be, and the less likely to make bad choices.

Keep in touch regularly. Kids will be more comfortable and forthcoming if you talk or text often. Sending a text message is a great way to get in touch any time of the day or night, and it's less expensive than a long-distance telephone call.

Another way to keep abreast of what's going on is to write or respond to your grandchild's blog. A blog, derived from the term "Web log," is a personal online journal. Blogs have become increasingly popular since their debut in 1994, and they can feature any subject. They might address controversial topics, such as politics, religion, and current events, but also fluffier fare about fashion and celebrities. They also function as personal diaries. Bloggers can change and update their sites at will, and there is no censoring.

Many free sites, such as www.livejournal.com, have interactive features that allow blog readers to write comments in response to the blogger's journal entries, and this can be a good way to keep in contact with faraway family and friends. Free blog services also keep an archive, so users can access their previous entries.

Some sites offer a "private" option that permits only certain readers to have access. However, for those who want their opinions and thoughts read by the general public, befriending unfamiliar visitors increases traffic to the site and exposure to the blogger's writing. In addition to the written entries, bloggers can post images (photos and artwork) and upload links to other sites.

Blogging is also a good way to get in touch with other people in your age group who share your interests. It's estimated that only 5 percent of bloggers on the Web are older than 50; however, blogster.com reports that 22 percent of their users are older than 50. Ronni Bennett, who runs a blog on aging called timegoesby.net, thinks the number of older bloggers will grow with time.

"When people quit working, their social group shrinks," he said. "Blogs enable people with similar interests to develop a new social group. Blogging also aids in keeping the brain sharp."

Visit www.blogger.com for more information, and www.createblog.com and blogster.com for ideas.

*Blogging is also a good way to get in touch with other people in your age group who share your interests. It's estimated that only 5 percent of bloggers on the Web are older than 50; however, blogster.com reports that 22 percent of their users are older than 50.*

## MAKING YOUR HOME SAFE FOR GRANDCHILDREN

To ensure that all goes well when the grandchildren visit you at home, it's critical to take precautions, particularly about water in bathtubs, swimming pools, lakes, and even buckets. Don't ever leave children unattended. If you must go, even for a moment, so should they, including from the tub. Children can drown in water as shallow as one inch if they can't lift their heads. Take care to fill the tub and turn off the water before putting in a child. To avoid burns, test the water to be sure it is not too hot and that the faucet has cooled off. Have supplies nearby— shampoo, soap, and towels—so that there is no reason to turn away, even for a moment.

Always insist that children wear U.S. Coast Guard-approved life vests—not floaties—particularly on boats or along the shoreline, where they could be washed away. Always keep rescue equipment (life preserver or shepherd's hook) and a telephone nearby.

Tender skin must be protected. Slather children in sunscreen with at least a 15 SPF sun blocker several times a day, even when it's cloudy. Carry a bottle in the car for unexpected stops. Outfit them in brimmed hats and sunglasses that will protect them (and also later become special souvenirs).

If you take children to a playground, don't let them wear anything with drawstrings, scarves, necklaces, belts, or backpacks, and avoid straps, such as those on a helmet. These things can get snagged on playground equipment and could cause injury. Choose an age-appropriate playground with soft surfaces, such as wood chips and shredded rubber, because falls on concrete, asphalt, or even packed dirt can lead to serious injury.

Make sure your grandchildren wear protective equipment, such as wrist guards and knee and elbow pads, when skating or riding a bicycle. Helmets reduce the risk of head injury by 85 percent, and they are required by law.

Lock up alcohol, medicine, household cleaning and garden chemicals, matches, lighters, candles, and all firearms. Keep knives, scissors, and hot plates out of reach. Put plug guards into sockets and around fires and heaters.

Keep a well-stocked first-aid kit and a fire extinguisher handy. More safety tips are available at www.safekids.org.

## TRAVELING WITH GRANDCHILDREN

Unlike in times past, when several generations worked side by side and lived under one roof or at least close-by, today's families are widely spread out. Airplanes and cars have made it possible to move to a city with better employment than a hometown might offer. This factor has certainly been a plus economically for the family, but easy mobility also has created a negative legacy.

Grandparents—who traditionally served as teachers, mentors, and role models for their grandchildren—have been left behind.

Stopping by Grandma's on the way home from school is rarely possible. Being actively involved in life experiences together is harder and less frequently possible, and relationships do not always have the opportunity to deepen. The loss can be profound.

Baby boomers are not content with superficial relationships. They want to spend time with their grandchildren and get to know them well. Older grandparents are healthier and more energetic than their predecessors, so they plan trips and vacations that include their grandchildren. They want to provide opportunities for bonding and creating wonderful memories, which is a more lasting inheritance than anything money can buy.

## Group Travel

Consider a trip specifically designed especially for grandchildren and their grandparents for greater ease, expert organization, and safety in numbers. All the activities will be kid-oriented, and opportunities will be available to interact with other grandparents. Traveling in a group offers assurance, and help will be available if problems occur.

Intergenerational vacations have become so common that new businesses have burgeoned to accommodate them. According to the Travel Industry Association of America, 30 percent of the U.S. leisure travelers who are grandparents have taken at least one vacation with their grandchildren. Kids—especially those aged 6–17—like to vacation with their grandparents. "Grandtravel" creates a special bond between the generations and creates unique memories.

A number of organizations offer a wide variety of packages and tours for grandparents and grandchildren, including:

- ▶ *Rascals in Paradise* has been providing worldwide vacation packages for families traveling with children of all ages since 1987. Visit www.rascalsinparadise.com.
- ▶ *Elderhostel*, which, as discussed earlier, provides outstanding educational travel experiences for people 55 and older, also offers

hundreds of intergenerational tours to domestic and international locations throughout the year. Packages range from short trips in the United States that cost less than $500 per person to costly multi-week international vacations. Packages include accommodations, most meals, transportation during the program, field trips, cultural events, and lectures, as well as gratuities and taxes. International programs also include airfare.

According to Elderhostel program guides, "Grandparents and grandkids can retrace the path of Lewis and Clark, explore the Everglades by canoe, learn about Irish mythology firsthand, bicycle through Germany and Austria, or choose from many other options, and the rates are the same for all ages!"

▶ *National Geographic* is also in the business of family adventures. You and your grandchildren can explore Alaska from a zodiac boat, safari in Kenya, or take photographs in Tonga. Their experts, who will know your destination well and are considered "family coordinators," design itineraries that include all the "can't miss spots," maximize the use of your time, and include kid activities. Visit www.nationalgeographicexpeditions.com for information.

▶ *Grandtravel.* For grandparents who want to treat their grandchildren to a deluxe travel experience, travel agencies such as Grandtravel offer first-class vacations to destinations around the world. Visit GrandTravel on the web at www.grandtrvl.com, or call 800-247-7651.

## FAMILY TRAVEL: EVERYBODY HOP IN!

If you decide not to join an organized group, but prefer a solo experience for your family, remember that you will need proper child restraints for your car, SUV, or RV; medical release forms signed by the parents, so that the children can be treated medically while in your care, if necessary; and a list of each child's medicines and prescriptions.

These last two items are required for group trips as well, but the tour company will provide assistance if you need it.

Leave a detailed itinerary with your grandchildren's parents, make sure you can be contacted, and allow the kids to contact their parents periodically. It's great fun for kids to share their experiences, because it helps lock in the memories. It's also comforting for kids to know they can chat with their parents whenever they want to.

Introduce the trip as a great adventure. Give your grandchildren a journal or diary, and a treasure box for their souvenirs. In addition to writing in the journal about their trip, they can include ticket stubs, postcards, restaurant menus, and photos. Encourage them to write a story about their adventures every day. It will make for great reading later.

Recreate your travel plan as a treasure map and teach your grandchildren to navigate. Choose some historic hotels and restaurants, and discuss what makes them special places. Dress up for dinner. They will never forget feeling so grown up, and you can use the opportunity to teach good manners and how to behave in more formal situations. If you can, avoid chain restaurants, and encourage trying new foods. Suggest a "two bites" policy—or, you could call it the "two bites" *game* for greater compliance.

Depending on the locale, you might take hikes and create a "treasure hunt" for souvenirs—a golden leaf, a pink rock, a feather, something old, something frilly, and an object with the name of the town on it are just a few examples.

Find a general store for fun and inexpensive souvenirs. On a family excursion to a quaint town in upstate New York, I took my children into the "dime store" (many towns still have them). I gave them a limit for what they could spend, but complete freedom to choose as they wished. All they wanted was a colorful plastic egg that was filled with Play Doh. Despite my urging to make additional choices, that was all they wanted. They played with it for hours every day in the car. Their choice was worth its weight in gold.

Visit the town's historic society. The people who work in local museums are a wealth of information about what makes their town unique. They can guide you about what to see and do during your visit. Often films, photographs, and artifacts of all sorts are on display. Taste a dish the town is known for, and have an ice cream cone in the soda shop. Many towns have them again because they are considered quaint, popular attractions.

Be on the lookout for children's museums, aquariums, zoos, water or amusement parks, and botanical or butterfly gardens. Kids love them all, but that doesn't mean you have to *do* them all. Be selective and pace yourself. You don't want to be too tired to enjoy the trip.

Play board or card games in the evening to unwind. However, try to follow the children's routine (hot baths, warm milk, regular bedtime) as best you can. Things will go much easier if they are expected to do what they always do. Then climb into bed and read some bedtime stories. What a great opportunity for cuddling.

## More Tips for a Smooth and Enjoyable Journey

▶ *Include your grandchildren in planning the trip.* They'll feel more invested in the adventure and will be more enthusiastic about participating in activities they have selected. Knowing what interests and excites your grandchildren can be the key to a successful trip.

▶ *Clear your travel itinerary with the child's parents.* They can provide tips about food preferences and nighttime routines that will be helpful. They will also give you information about allergies, necessary medications, and medical insurance provisions.

▶ *Before your big trip, try a shorter excursion first,* such as an overnight stay in your home or a weekend away.

▶ *If the kids have never tried room service in a hotel, order in one evening.*

▶ *Set spending limits.* Decide prior to the trip how much the children can spend on snacks, activities, and souvenirs.

▶ *Give each child a disposable camera.* If you are going to beach locations, an underwater camera makes for some beautiful and unique photos. Take a digital camera to avoid having to buy film. Remember to take multiple memory cards that are large enough to accommodate the hundreds of photos everyone will want to take.

▶ *Don't plan every minute of the vacation.* Leave room in your schedule for quiet time. Take books, games, and puzzles to create peaceful moments, and so the children will have something to do when waiting in line, in restaurants, or while driving.

▶ *Have an end-of-trip party* after you get home that includes a dinner with the food from one of the states or countries you visited, a slide show of photographs, and a personalized scrapbook for each child. In traveling with your grandchildren, you will have created an unequaled memory that will bond you to them forever.

## ROAD TRIP FUN

In case you've forgotten how you passed the time during a long road trip with your own children, here is a short list of fun and educational games. Consider the age of the children when deciding what to play. You don't want to frustrate them with a game that they don't understand. Singing along is great fun, too, so bring their favorite tapes or CDs.

▶ *The Synonym/Antonym Game.* Begin with the eldest in the car. This person says a word, and each person who follows says a word that means either the same or the opposite of that word.

▶ *The Build-a-Sentence Game.* The eldest (among the adults) begins with a word, and then each player adds a word to make a meaningful sentence. Don't let the sentence end. Tip: Run-on sentences are the rule, not the offense, in this game.

▶ *The Build-a-Story Game.* Beginning with the eldest again (then taking turns going first), and proceeding clockwise through the players in the vehicle, each participant adds a sentence to make an original story. It might be whacky, scary, or fairy-princess-happily-ever-after fantastical. Each sentence has to have relevance to the story. Tip: If you can, make a recording! This game might be easier for the four- or five-year olds than the Build-a-Sentence game. Encourage their efforts and help them if needed. Make your own set of rules for this game, such as whether or not you will allow run-on sentences.

▶ *Spell-a-Word Rules.* Beginning with the eldest in the car, say a letter. Proceed around the vehicle with each player adding a letter to spell a real word of more than three letters. The trick is to always have a real word in mind when it's your turn. Players can challenge one another if they think another player does not have a real word in mind. For instance, it comes to you and your child has just said "v" to the end of the series "abse." If he doesn't have a valid word in mind, you win. If he does, he wins. The goal is to keep the word going. If you end it, you lose.

▶ *The License Plate Game.* In this game, the children have to create a list of the states they notice before anyone else. When they see a new state on a license plate, they call "dibs" and then write down the state's name, color of the plate, and symbol. The one who has the most states at the end of the trip wins.

▶ *Bury-the-Cows Rules.* All players are divided into either the right- or left-hand side of the vehicle. Players count the cows on their side (or horses, sheep, goats, ducks, or camels—whatever animal is likely to be found in the region). When one side or the other sees a cemetery (or body of water such as a river, pond, or lake) the other side's herd is lost, and they must build up their herd again. This game continues as long as you like, with the winning team having the biggest herd.

▶ *The "First" Game.* When you're approaching a town, everyone has to be on alert for the first of everything—the first gas station, the first McDonalds, the first amusement park, the first fire station, the first police officer, etc. Whoever sees these things first gets a point. This game encourages the kids to really look at their surroundings.

## Discounted Destinations

Grandparents—if they're senior citizens—and kids can reap the benefits of their age group with discounted prices for fares, tour costs, entrance fees, lodging, and food. These discounts also apply to resorts and cruises, and everything is included—accommodations, food, and organized activities for kids. There are all kinds of places to visit, and you never have to leave the property to have the perfect vacation.

Cruises offer fabulous food (and *you* don't have to pick up the tab), lively entertainment and activities, a chance to relax, and the opportunity to see a variety of port cities. For general information about some of the well-known cruise lines, call Cruises Only at 888-278-4737, or check out www.cruiseline.com. The Resource section at the end of the book lists some favorite kid-friendly cruise lines and popular resorts.

## Gifts for Grandkids

Giving gifts is one way to express love. Unlike parents, who might worry about spoiling a child with too many things, grandparents are fairly free to give what they like to a grandchild. The gifts need not be expensive to be special and remembered forever. For me, it was the crisp one-dollar bill that my grandfather gave my siblings, my cousins, and me at the end of every weekly visit to my grandparents' home. I don't remember any other gift they ever gave me, although there were many, but I remember those dollars vividly and with complete pleasure, because it reminds me so much of him.

In *How to Build the Grandma Connection*, Susan V. Bosak (The Legacy Project at www.legacyproject.org) suggests "practical ideas, inspiration, and wisdom you need to build loving, rewarding, lifelong relationships with your grandchildren." In the following excerpt from her book, she addresses the variables to consider before buying just the right gift.

The most important cautions are: don't overwhelm your grandchildren with too many gifts; don't try to buy their affection; don't go against their parents' wishes; and never buy a big gift or one that will require special care or arrangements (such as a pet or a trip) without first consulting the parents. You may also want to stay away from clothing, since children's sizes and tastes are so variable.

Gifts can stimulate your grandchild's imagination, entertain, educate, or simply offer pure delight. In general, there are two kinds of gifts: formal gifts for birthdays and holidays; and "little things" you give just to make your grandchild feel special.

The following is a list of her suggestions for how to handle specific gift-giving challenges:

▶ *Toys.* Children today have so many toys, many of which quickly become discarded or broken. Try to give your grandchildren toys that have lasting value or can be used to be creative; for example, art supplies, building sets, board games, or a microscope. The more flexible and unstructured the toy, the more lasting it will tend to be.

It's okay to indulge your grandchild once in a while with an extravagant or "fad" gift they just "have to have." But consult with their parents first to make sure they don't have any strong objections.

Try to break the toy stereotypes. Don't just give dolls to girls and trucks to boys. There's one woman I know whose parents would never buy her a train set—despite her pleas for one, Christmas after Christmas. Finally, her Grandma took her seriously and bought her the set she wanted so badly. Today, that woman is 47 years old, and she still has and cherishes that train set.

► *Get creative.* Gifts are limited only by your imagination. Use these ideas to get you started:

  – *Play detective.* What are your grandchild's interests and blooming talents? Give gifts that encourage and support them; for example, tickets to events, plays, and concerts; creative lessons (such as ballet or martial arts); musical instruments; sports equipment; a magazine subscription; posters or paintings; calendars; videos; or computer software.

  – *Buy your grandchild things "big kids" need,* such as a radio, clock, camera, desk, bookcase, or bags for carrying things to school, for sports, or for travel.

  – *Books are always in style,* and they won't break.

  – *Your junk mail can be a source of stickers, labels, and pages* that can be painted or colored. Wrap them up with a bow, and they become something fun.

  – *Plan a treasure hunt* with clues your grandchild can follow to find items hidden around your house.

  – *Give your grandchild a disposable camera* with a list of places and things they can find and photograph.

► *Collectibles.* Help your grandchild start a collection and then add to it over time. It might be cards (baseball to dinosaur), rocks, stamps, coins, comic books, miniatures, or figurines. You can give sticker and sticker book sets to younger children. For example, give your grandchild an animal sticker book and buy packets of animal stickers over time for her to stick in the right spot and learn about animals. Whatever the collection, it becomes a common interest you can share.

► *Playful gifts.* One woman told me that during her four years in college she looked forward to letters from her grandmother more than anyone else. They always contained a little "surprise"—perhaps a stick of gum, a cartoon clipped from the newspaper, a funny sticker, or a lucky coin. You can give or mail your grandchild a little something every once in a while as a surprise. It's not the gift itself that's important, but the connection it makes, because it says, "I'm thinking about you."

Send something small and inexpensive, perhaps once a month or so (but don't feel pressured). You can start when your grandchild is around 3 years old. Craft shops and "dollar" stores are great places for these kinds of little gifts. Be creative and imaginative. You might send a finger puppet, a small stencil, funny socks, a balloon with a message on it ("Blow up this balloon to read a surprise message from Grandma"), a musical toothbrush, a pen in the shape of a snake (there are some wild things in dollar stores!), or even a magazine ad or photo cut up like a puzzle. You can also send things your grandchild can experiment with, such as a magnifying glass, magnet, or flower and vegetable seeds.

Sometimes it's a nice idea to enclose a note with playful gifts suggesting things your grandchild can do. For example: "Here's a magnifying glass that's especially for you! If you hold it up to your eye and look through it, things will look bigger. Take it around the house and look closely at the wooden railing along the stairs, the carpet, a banana peel, a raisin. What do you see? Look at your brother's nose. Does it look bigger? Let me know what else you see with your magnifying glass."

▶ *Handmade gifts.* Something handmade makes a special gift in the present, and it can become a treasured keepsake over the years. You might make your grandchild a quilt, a special blanket, a sweater or scarf, a fancy T-shirt, a stuffed doll or bear, or doll clothes. If sewing, knitting, or needlework is new to you, start with a kit from a needlework or craft shop.

If you don't have the time or skill to make your grandchild "traditional" things, try your hand at more playful handmade crafts. It's the thought and creativity you put into it that counts. For example, make a picture out of pennies stuck to a sheet of colored cardboard (you can even spell out your grandchild's name). Your grandchild can admire the picture for a while, and then put the coins in his piggy bank. Another idea is to make shapes and animals out of the fuzzy "wire twisties" available in craft stores. You might make a giraffe out of a yellow twistie, and then send it to your grandchild with another yellow twistie to playfully "challenge" her to make the same animal.

▶ *Money.* Money is always welcome, even in small amounts. You just don't want it to be the only gift you give, or use it as a way to "buy" your grandchildren's affection. My grandmother would often let me have the change after I went to the store for her, or she would give me a dollar when I helped her with something. It didn't happen all the time, and I didn't perceive it as payment for services rendered. I just felt special when she gave me "a little something" that was all my own.

You can be creative with money. A roll of quarters can even be magic. Another twist is to give your grandchild a sum of money with the proviso that he must give it to a charity of his own choosing. This can spark some good conversations with older grandchildren, teach them about helping others, and help them think about what they value and why.

You might decide to do more for your grandchild as they start to get older, such as buying savings bonds or stocks, or contributing to your grandchild's college education. Instead of waiting until you're gone, you might also consider letting your older grandchildren know that you have money available for big wishes or needs, such as helping to buy a car or getting special medical treatment.

A word of caution: If you give money to your grandchildren, or to your adult children for your grandchildren, be careful about putting restrictions on its use. If you can afford it, and it's coming from your heart, just give it—with the assumption that it will be used wisely. To do otherwise is to put a strain on your family relationships.

▶ *Time.* Time is the greatest gift of all. Time "coupons" are a creative way for both you and your grandchild to anticipate a fun, shared experience. They also give your grandchild power in "redeeming" the coupon. You might give coupons for baking cookies, reading a story, going shopping, or learning how to do woodworking.

▶ *"Thank-you" notes.* Parents have an important role to play in encouraging bonds between their children and grandparents. One of the easiest ways to do this is to help children write a simple "thank-you" note for a gift from a grandparent. So many grandparents I talk to say this is THE biggest complaint they have—they never get a thank-you note. They often don't even know if a grandchild has received their gift safely, let alone whether or not they like it. If grandparents don't get feedback, how can they know what to give grandchildren?

> *Parents have an important role to play in encouraging bonds between their children and grandparents. One of the easiest ways to do this is to help children write a simple "thank-you" note for a gift from a grandparent. So many grandparents I talk to say this is THE biggest complaint they have—they never get a thank-you note.*

The note doesn't have to be fancy or long. It can just acknowledge receipt of the gift; have a line describing what the grandchild likes about the gift, or what they're going to do with it, and then end with "thank you" and "I love you."

Learning to say "thank you" teaches children an important social skill, and makes grandparents feel loved and appreciated. It gets a two-way communication going.

What can a grandparent do to encourage thank-you notes? Talk to your adult children about how important acknowledgment is to you. You can also use this as an opportunity to teach them a social grace. Explain that you want to hear from them about what they liked or didn't like about a gift. Be persistent in your communication, without anger or criticism.

As a hint or reminder, some grandparents enclose a "fill-in-the-blanks" card they write out for grandchildren to return to them. Another good idea is to set an example yourself—acknowledge and thank your grandchildren for something they've sent or given you, or even for a phone call.

## Gifts Create Family Bonds

Giving gifts should be an act of love, a way to make the recipient feel special, and an important legacy from one generation to another. I treasure the things my grandmother gave me—her silver tea service, an ornate vase she bought on her trip to Italy, a gold bracelet, and the beautiful bowl she loved best for mixing the ingredients of the meals we prepared together.

She gave me these things ceremonially, and with a detailed description of their history. These were no longer just "things" she had once bought. She chose to give me these treasures so that I would know how special I was to her. They became symbols of the love she had for me. Now, each time I look at her special gifts, I think of my grandmother and the love we shared. They are sweet reminders of our precious relationship.

We generally spend the first half of our life collecting things and the second half giving these same things away. Do it thoughtfully, and the objects you've bought throughout the years will give you enjoyment a second time around—and they will also give others something to remember you by later.

*We generally spend the first half of our life collecting things and the second half giving these same things away. Do it thoughtfully, and the objects you've bought throughout the years will give you enjoyment a second time around—and they will also give others something to remember you by later.*

Consider these tips when deciding what to give the generation that will carry your memory in their hearts and share stories about you with *their* children:

▶ *Give keepsakes* that will elicit a memory—a photograph of a special outing, a hat you once wore that you allowed your grandchild to play with, an important piece of jewelry that they should take care of, a candy dish, a perfume bottle. When they look at those objects, they will be reminded of you and the moment the gifts were given.

▶ *Pass down gifts you've received to create a living legacy*—a handmade tablecloth from your mother, a diary your aunt kept, rare books that your uncle collected, or an antique table passed from one family member to the next. These gifts can serve to connect the generations and give children a context within which to live their lives. Our feeling of value and pride initially comes from our family. We feel important when we have a place in history, even if it is only within our own family.

▶ *Take time to identify objects in your home* that you are not yet ready to pass on but want others to know about. Place tags underneath the objects that include stories about them, and dates and place of purchase, if you know them. Say why they are important and to whom they should be given. This act will simplify what happens after you pass on, alleviating others of a difficult decision-making process.

▶ *Create a family tree.* It's important for people to know where and from whom they've come, even though families are mobile today and members can be scattered all over globe. Older members of the family eventually pass away, and the keepers of the information are often gone before someone decides documentation of the family history should be done. If you have not secured this important information before then, your job will be far more complicated, but not impossible. Visit www.ancestry.com or www.myheritage.com/familytree for help in doing the research and www.smartdraw.com for creating the document. Use full names, dates and places of birth, photos if you have them, and descriptions of the people. Then make copies and send them to all your relatives. In this way, you will have become the storyteller for the history of your family and passed on an unequaled legacy. Your grandchildren will enjoy the detective work involved and be proud of the results, and everyone in the family will love you for it.

▶ *Mark important moments.* Buy and save the newspaper the day of a grandchild's birth. Celebrate the birth by making a video or tape recording. Tell the child about your family, what your life is like, how much you love them, and any words of wisdom. Give it to the parents with a note that it's not to be played until a birthday when the child is old enough to appreciate it. If all the family members are still available, you will have quite an important treat waiting. If someone is no longer with you, that person and their love will have been documented for posterity. The best thing I did was to interview my grandmother and father on video about their lives. I documented the details of both sides of our family history, and I also captured forever their personhood—their look, voice, and mannerisms—for generations to come. I'm sorry I didn't do this with my mother. I thought I had time because she was younger. I was wrong.

▶ *Create rituals*—family traditions that everyone can depend on—special foods for every holiday dinner, a yearly family reunion, a letter of gratitude and love sent each year to your loved ones, a regular outing to the park for a picnic on the first day of spring, or a family excursion each year to the first game of the season of the sport you all like the most. Each Christmas, I gave my children a new ornament to hang on the tree that represented whatever they most loved that year. One day they will have their own trees, and all those ornaments will be gifted to them again. You can easily do this with your grandchildren. Be sure to put their names on each ornament and the year given, so there won't be confusion later.

It doesn't matter what the rituals are; just make sure you have some. They bond a family together and create security. In an uncertain world, it's critical for family members to believe there are people and events on which they can always depend.

## CONSIDER PUTTING GIFTS TO GRANDCHILDREN IN A TRUST

If your income provides adequately for your needs—and you have discretionary funds that you would like to give others—consider putting money aside for your grandchildren. It will benefit both them and you.

An individual can give a grandchild up to $12,000 a year without having to report the gift, so there is no tax consequence. A couple can give as much as $24,000 to each grandchild. This is in addition to paying for health care or school costs to an institution of higher learning, if you should choose to participate in the support of their education in this way.

Putting money in trust for your grandchildren is a good strategy for reducing the size of your estate and the inheritance taxes due on that estate when you die. However, certain requirements must be met by the individuals who are doing the gifting, so it is wise to have an attorney set up the appropriate trusts for your financial situation. Costs are involved in hiring a trust attorney, so be sure to shop around for one with a good reputation and a reasonable price. Consider an attorney who is an elderlaw specialist.

According to www.elderlawanswers.com, "With the help of your attorney, you can draft a trust that reflects your express wishes about when the income and principal will be available to the grandchild, and even how the funds will be spent."

Transferring funds into a trust offers the following benefits:

▶ You can reduce the size of your estate by transferring up to $12,000 (in 2007) into each trust you create for each grandchild. No gift taxes will be due in connection with the transfers.

▶ Although the trust owns the assets, you control the assets, and you can decide what type of investments to make.

▶ Income earned by the trust from amounts that you've deposited will not be taxed to you. The trust pays the taxes.

▶ Amounts deposited in trust, and the income earned from those funds, will be used for the benefit of your grandchildren.

▶ You can terminate the trust at an age that you specify.

## 529 Accounts

Named for Section 529 of the Internal Revenue Code, this type of account enables you to reduce your taxable estate while delegating funds for the higher education of a grandchild (or any other family member). Monies contributed to such accounts are invested to pay for a grandchild's college tuition, room and board, or other expenses.

Under the tax law passed in 2001, the earnings from these accounts are tax-free beginning in 2002—previously they were taxable to the beneficiary when used to pay for college. You can contribute up to $12,000 (in 2007) per year ($24,000 for a couple) to 529 accounts without incurring a gift tax. If you prefer, you can contribute up to $60,000 ($120,000 for a married couple) in the first year of a 5-year period, as long as no additional gifts are made to that same beneficiary over the 5 years.

A 529 account is a quick way of getting a sizable amount of money out of your taxable estate. However, if you die within the 5-year period, the portion of the contribution that was allocated to the years following your death would be again considered as part of your estate.

An additional benefit of these accounts is that the donors can take the money back later if needed, although a penalty of 10 percent of earnings would have to be paid. However, the power to control the assets means that the savings in a 529 account can be counted as an asset under Medicaid rules, in the event the donor requires long-term care.

If the grandchild uses the funds for any purpose other than higher education, the earnings are taxed as ordinary income to the account owner (you), and a 10 percent penalty is assessed on investment gains.

A 529 account generally does not affect a child's eligibility for financial aid, because you are the account owner. This change may increase a student's chances for financial aid, because qualified withdrawals will no longer be considered income to the student.

Additionally, you can change beneficiaries at any time, as long as the new beneficiary is a member of the original beneficiary's family. The tax law enacted in 2001 expanded the list of family members to include the first cousin of the original beneficiary.

Most states permit, or are planning to permit, 529 account plans, and many investment firms offer them as tax- and estate-planning vehicles for their clients. The website www.savingforcollege.com compares the different state plans.

## IRAs

You can make contributions to your grandchildren's regular, Roth, or Educational IRAs. Roth IRAs can be a particularly good way to help a grandchild create a financial nest egg.

The amounts contributed to an IRA account are not tax-deductible, but the accumulated earnings can be withdrawn beginning at age 59½ completely tax-free. Some conditions for withdrawal exist.

Tax-free compounding can add up, and your beneficiary needs to understand this. For example, if a 15-year-old contributes $2,000 to a Roth IRA today, the investment (with a 10 percent annual return) will be worth $146,000 when he turns 60.

The other advantage of setting up such an account is that first-time homebuyers can withdraw up to $10,000 tax-free after the account has been established for a period of 5 years. If Roth IRAs are used to pay college tuition, no withdrawal penalties will apply.

Participating in this way can be an opportunity to teach your grandchildren fiscal responsibility, how to save money for their future (even their own retirement), the principles of investing, and how to avoid debt.

## Savings Bonds

United States Savings Bonds are the most widely held type of security. Bonds increase in value monthly and interest is compounded semi-annually.

The interest is free from state and local taxes, and federal income tax is deferred until you redeem the bonds. You can reap special tax benefits if bonds are redeemed to pay for college expenses, after you've met certain eligibility requirements.

Series EE and the new Series I Bonds make great gifts for grandchildren. Series EE Bonds sell for half their face value. The bond denominations range from $50 to $10,000. If they are not redeemed when they mature, they will continue to earn interest for up to 30 years.

Series I Savings Bonds come in denominations ranging from $50 to $10,000 and are issued at face value. The earnings rate, adjusted semiannually, is a combination of a fixed interest rate at the time of purchase and the rate of inflation. These bonds have a 30-year life.

Current rates for both the EE and I Bond are available by calling 1-800-4USBond. Additional information on U.S. Savings Bonds can be found at www.savingsbonds.gov. Savings bonds can now be ordered directly online with a credit card.

The joys and rewards of being a grandparent are many, and well worth the effort. Whether you live next door—or across the country—you can create beautiful memories for your grandchildren that will last *their* lifetime, and beyond.

# Part III

Take Charge of Your Life

# Age-proofing Your Home

## *Create a Safe Environment*

*Dear Ageless:*

*I'm interested in making the kitchen safer for myself and my mom, who is struggling with arthritis and dementia. What do you suggest?*

*Cookin' with Fire*

*Dear Cookin' with Fire:*

*The kitchen is the most dangerous room in the house, particularly for those who are busy, frail, or absent-minded. Almost 1 million injuries and deaths occur each year because of unsafe kitchen environments, including accidents involving forgotten pots left on the stovetop, scalding water from faucets, gas leaks from an extinguished pilot light, and electrical shocks.*

*According to The Home Safety Council, "Research shows that most home fires begin in the kitchen. To help keep the risk of injuries low in your kitchen, keep oven mitts and pan lids easily accessible and learn the preferred method for extinguishing a pan fire. Understand how to best handle different types of fires that can occur while cooking and be aware that, in many cases,* evacuating the home is your best defense. Once you get out of the house, it's important to stay out. Do not go back inside for any reason.

Pan Fires: Always keep a potholder, oven mitt, and lid handy. If a small grease fire starts in a pan, put on an oven mitt and smother the flames by carefully sliding the lid over the pan. Sliding a lid over a burning pan is a relatively safe way to extinguish a small grease fire. Placing the lid from front to back will limit your exposure to the flames and scalding grease. With the lid covering the flames, it is easier to turn off the burner. As long as the lid stays on, the oxygen is cut off, and the fire can die out naturally. This procedure is widely recommended by safety authorities and is preferred over portable fire extinguishers, which if used improperly could push burning grease and flames off the pan and spread the fire. Baking soda can also be used to extinguish a small pan fire; however the user risks greater exposure to the heat, flames, and scalding grease. Do not use baking powder because it can burn and would actually add fuel to the fire.

Don't remove the lid until it is completely cool. Never pour water on a grease fire and never try to move or carry a burning pan, as you can be severely burned by hot grease and can easily spread the fire.

Oven Fires: Turn off the heat and keep the door closed to prevent flames from burning you and your clothing. Call the fire department to report the incidence so that firefighters can check for possible flame spread.

Toaster Oven or Microwave Fires: Keep the door closed and unplug the appliance if you can safely reach the receptacle. Call the fire department to report the fire. Have the appliance serviced before you use it again, or replace it.

Using a Portable Fire Extinguisher: If you know how to safely use a portable fire extinguisher, you may be able to put out a small, contained fire, such as a toaster oven or trash fire.

*Always call the fire department before fighting the fire, and make sure everyone else has left the building  Never let the fire get positioned between you and the exit."*

*Visit www.homesafetycouncil.org for other important tips and guidelines.*

*Ageless*

Home safety is important for us all, but it becomes a primary concern as we grow older. Kitchens, baths, hallways, and stairs can be the source of problems.

## SAFETY IN THE KITCHEN

▶ *Determine if your kitchen meets general safety standards.* Appliances should work well, be clean, and be disconnected when not in use. Electrical cords should not be frayed, cracked, or trailing across the floor or worktop (buy curly cords), and outlet extensions that accommodate several plugs should not be used.

▶ *Install circuit breakers to provide overload protection.* Use ground-fault circuit interrupters to protect against electric shock, and equip gas stoves with an automatic cut-off in the event of flame failure. Always buy coffeepots, teakettles, and irons with automatic shut-offs.

▶ *Set the hot water heater's thermostat at 110°F,* and install a single-lever faucet that balances water temperature to prevent burns. Floors should be non-slip. Avoid loose rugs, and store heavy objects on bottom shelves.

▶ *Install pull-out shelves inside cabinets and lazy Susans* (swivel plates) in corner cabinets. Install handles on cabinet doors rather than knobs (easier to grab).

▶ *Improve lighting to prevent accidents*—for example, from knife misuse and medicine mix-ups—and so that spills are more visible.

Reduce glare with frosted bulbs, increase wattage in over-the-countertop lights, and install fixtures under cabinets to illuminate countertop work spaces.

▶ *Keep flammable items (including towels and curtains) away from the stovetop and oven.* Avoid wearing clothing with loose or long sleeves when cooking.

▶ *Install a smoke detector, and have a fire blanket and extinguisher immediately accessible.* Hang a list of emergency numbers next to the telephone. Visit the U.S. Consumer Product Safety Commission at www.cpsc.gov/cpscpub for more recommendations and valuable publications.

After you implement these changes in your home, suggest doing the same in your parents' home. Take the time to discuss safety measures with them. Depending on your parents' age and physical condition, you might also want to practice with them what to do in the event of an accident in the home.

## Safety in the Bathroom

The bathroom is the second most dangerous room in the house. Smooth surfaces, glass and mirrors, soap and water, and the small size of a bathroom can spell disaster, particularly for older people. You need to take precautions against falls, burns, poisons, drowning, and electrical injuries.

The ideal bathroom location for someone who needs to use a walker or wheelchair—or who may need one in the future—is on the first floor. Make sure the bathroom includes:

▶ A door that swings out, providing good access for the walker or chair and allowing access to a fallen person blocking the door

▶ A 32-inch doorway without a sill, and with a 5-foot turning radius

- ▶ Rounded-edge cabinetry and countertops with knee space to accommodate a wheelchair
- ▶ A slip-resistant floor of matte-finished vinyl, textured tile, or a low-pile carpet; no throw-rugs or bathmats
- ▶ A roll-in shower with tempered or shatterproof-glazed glass doors

This can be an expensive proposition unless the accessible bathroom is installed at the time a house is built. In many cases, an existing bathroom can be made quite accessible with some fairly simple changes:

- ▶ *Install non-skid, adhesive strips in the shower and bathtub,* and institutional-grade, stainless steel grab bars for solid support in the bath and near a toilet. Have a professional do the installation. It's imperative that grab bars remain stationary when someone pulls on them.
- ▶ *Use a portable, waterproof, non-slip shower chair and a hand-held showerhead,* for people who cannot safely stand.
- ▶ *Hang a liquid soap and shampoo dispenser to minimize bending.* Avoid using soap cakes, because they can slip from the hand and create a fall hazard.
- ▶ *Wipe up spills from shower or tub immediately,* or carpet the entire bathroom to avoid slips and falls. If you choose carpeting, clean it regularly and replace it periodically because germs, mold, and mildew will grow more readily.
- ▶ *Avoid using bath oil in the tub or shower* because it will leave a slippery residue.
- ▶ *Install a heat lamp in the ceiling* to maintain a warm temperature in the bathroom. This is especially important for people who have rheumatoid arthritis.
- ▶ *Avoid using electrical equipment in the bathroom as much as possible.* Water contact with this equipment can cause an electrical shock.

▶ *Install an adjustable toilet seat* or make sure the seat is 18 inches from the floor for easier transfer from a wheelchair. Some people do not find the higher "disabled" toilet height comfortable, so be sure that everyone who will use the bathroom is consulted during the decision-making process.

▶ *Attach or place toilet frames, arm rests, or commodes* around the toilet.

▶ *Insulate exposed pipes,* and mount a single-lever, touchless or push-button faucet with temperature and volume controls to prevent burns. If possible, set the water heater at 110°F to avoid scalds.

▶ *Do not keep medications in the bathroom.* Organization and careful dispensing of medications is difficult, and the moisture and heat can be damaging. Be sure that toiletries and medicines are stored separately from household cleansers.

▶ *Increase lighting for the vision-impaired.* Rocker light switches and levered door and drawer pulls are crucial for people with arthritic hands and weakened muscles. Install a night-light and easy-to-reach telephone or emergency call button. Keep a key just outside the bathroom door in case a person inside the bathroom is unable to unlock the door.

Visit www.carepathways.com and www.senioremporium.com for more information on bathroom safety and for ordering useful equipment. See also, http://www.usfa.fema.gov.

## CREATE A BEDROOM THAT ACCOMMODATES *YOUR* NEEDS

▶ *Put a bright lamp that cannot be easily knocked over next to the bed,* or locate the bed next to a light switch. This will enable an older person to find her way to the bathroom at night.

▶ *Put a stable night stand next to the bed,* so that glasses and other necessary items will be within easy reach.

▶ *Put a phone on the bedside table* for frail, elderly people who are able to use it. It will be extremely helpful in an emergency, and just knowing it's there will relieve anxiety.

▶ *Use a night light,* so that visibility is good during the night.

▶ *Keep clear pathways around the bed,* to the door, and to the bathroom.

▶ *Remove casters on beds, tables, and chairs.* Unintended movement of furniture that might be used for support can result in a fall.

▶ *Mount a grab bar, railing, or rope in the hallways* if the bedroom is not easily accessible to the bathroom or living areas. Heavy pieces of furniture can also be strategically placed to support a frail person in moving from room to room.

▶ *Use a hot water bottle for warmth at bedtime.* Avoid using heating pads and electric blankets when sleeping. Older people are less sensitive to heat and may inadvertently become overheated or burned.

▶ *Designate smoking areas.* If anyone in the household smokes, arrange a specific, safe place in the house where smoking is allowed. Discourage smoking in bed or while sitting on upholstered furniture.

▶ *Adjust the bed height,* so that the older person can get in and out of bed comfortably.

▶ *See that storage spaces and needed items are within easy reach* and that there is enough light to find things.

## Adjustable Beds

A good night's sleep is crucial for optimum health, but it might become more of a problem as we grow older. An adjustable bed that elevates both the back and legs offers many advantages. It minimizes the gaps between the body and the mattress to alleviate pressure points and back and neck pain, breathing disorders improve with better air exchange and reduced snoring, and problems such as acid reflux disease, heartburn, arthritis, and edema (fluid accumulation in the legs and feet) can be relieved.

Adjustable beds—manual, semi-electric, and fully electric—vary among manufacturers. Be sure that the frame is all-steel with riveted joints (no pieces to come loose) and that it has the desired amount of lift and height for transferring a frail person easily to a walker or wheelchair. The electric motor should be sealed to keep out dust and dirt, and so that it won't need lubrication; the bed control should be wireless and lighted.

The mattress can be soft to ultra-firm, and it can be made with traditional innerspring construction (double offset coil is best) or with either high-density foam or less-expensive latex for greatest body conformity. Look for a stain-resistant cover or one that is detachable and can be put in the washing machine.

Consider added features such as guard rails, heater, and massager. Test the level of noise when using various options. Read the warranty carefully, and compare costs for shipping and handling.

If the person who will use the bed has both Medicare Part A and B, he might be entitled to a "rent-to-own" bed. However, it can only be a hospital bed, and a physician must certify medical necessity. Visit www.usfa.fema.gov for more information.

## GENERAL SAFETY TIPS

▶ *Keep a list of telephone numbers to call in case of an emergency* (911, doctors, relatives) *near the phone in* large, *readable type or handwriting.*

▶ *Check all electrical cords and replace those that show signs of wear.*

▶ *Install adequate electrical outlets to prevent overloading circuits.*

▶ *Avoid multiple extension cords* or electric cords stretched across open areas or doorways, and use coiled cords wherever possible.

▶ *Use non-skid wax to clean uncarpeted floors.*

▶ *Use rubber-backed throw rugs*, or place non-skid strips on backs of rugs.

▶ *Use bright lighting* that is even throughout the house or apartment.

▶ *Be sure the doors can be unlocked from the outside in case of an emergency.* This is especially important in the bathroom and bedroom.

▶ *Put smoke detectors and fire extinguishers in appropriate places* throughout the house or apartment, including the kitchen and bedroom. Check smoke detector batteries twice a year.

▶ *Draw up and practice an evacuation plan in case of fire or other emergency.*

## SAFETY TIPS FOR STAIRS, PATHWAYS, AND GARDENS

▶ *Place brightly colored, non-skid strips on the edge of steps* to prevent falls.

▶ *Light stairways, hallways, and indoor and outdoor pathways* brightly and evenly.

▶ *Remove any object that juts out from stairways or pathways*, including coat hooks, low light fixtures, and shelves.

▶ *Check steps and walkways for holes, cracks, and splinters*; make needed repairs.

▶ *Consider using ramps, even for people who do not use wheelchairs.* They can be easier to negotiate.

▶ *Use smooth but slip-resistant handrails along stairways.*

▶ *Avoid placing sharp rocks or objects along garden pathways.* Keep hoses away from walkways. Store garden equipment between uses.

▶ *Use a cane or walker* if unsteady gait is a problem.

▶ *Wear sunglasses and a hat or cap* while out-of-doors to help prevent glare and protect against the sun.

▶ *Put reflector tape on shoes and clothing* that will be worn while walking in twilight or the evening. Orange or yellow reflectorized garments can be worn after dark.

## FOOTWEAR

▶ *Choose shoes that are as lightweight as possible.* They should be flexible and form-fitting. Natural materials, including suede and leather, are cooler than manmade materials such as plastic and nylon. Shoes with Velcro™ straps are easier to put on and take off.

▶ *Choose soles made of material that grips the floor,* such as corrugated rubber. Leather, wood, cork, or crepe soled shoes may crack and cause falls.

▶ *Consider having your feet checked for fallen arches,* which can contribute to difficulty walking and low back pain. A molded insert in the shoe may be the answer for a pain-free gait.

## ASSISTIVE DEVICES

### General Tips

▶ *Buy reaching tools* that make grabbing things easier, even from a sitting position or a wheelchair.

▶ *Invest in a hands-free can opener, a jar opener, and a pill bottle opener* for people who have trouble gripping or who have arthritis.

▶ *Invest in a good cane.* Canes allow for greater balance and also widen the base of support. Although they can be bought in drugstores and over the Internet, they must still be fitted to the height of the user to achieve comfortable use. Visit www.fashionablecanes.com/caneinfo.htm#fit for information.

▶ *Use a walker when weight-bearing is a problem;* walkers must be fitted properly by a physical therapist.

### Wheelchairs

Losing something as precious as our mobility and independence is a major event, and it's often accompanied by anger, sadness, and depression. When this happens, we have to recognize and accept that our body is not only aging, but ailing as well. So it's important to understand, empathize, and be patient during this process.

Wheelchairs fall into two broad types: (1) manual chairs powered by the user or by someone pushing, and (2) motorized (power wheelchairs or scooters). Both types provide mobility, but each type has advantages and disadvantages. Manual wheelchairs, particularly those that are collapsible for easy transport, aren't as sturdy and don't offer as much independence; power wheelchairs are heavy and require more maintenance.

Before making a decision regarding a wheelchair purchase, consider these factors:

▶ The chair width should be narrow enough to pass through the home, but wide enough to accommodate the user's hips, with 2 inches extra on each side.

▶ The chair frame should be designed for durability—a folding chair is less sturdy because of its moving parts, but a rigid-frame chair is harder to transport.

▶ The chair should have easy-to-apply brakes, a safety-lock system, and come with a warranty.

▶ The cushion is an important component of the wheelchair, and it should be prescribed separately by a medical professional. It should be made from a comfortable material, such as vinyl, cloth, or leather.

Cost is a consideration, and a physician must write a *durable medical equipment* (DME) prescription for a wheelchair. Medicare Part B (for those over 65 or with certain disabilities) will cover 80 percent of the approved amount, not including the deductible, if the DME is reasonable and necessary in the treatment of an injury or illness, and the chair will be used in the home. Call Medicare at 800-633-4227 for information.

If the chair is not covered by Medicare Part B, other sources of wheelchair funding include Medicaid and the Veterans Administration. You can also try calling Wishes on Wheels at 800-535-3063 for help in acquiring a power wheelchair.

## Make Your Home Secure

► *Get a security check-up.* Most local police departments have literature about how to make your home secure. Some police departments have officers who will check your home for potential problems. Call and ask if they do inspections, and then implement any recommendations they make.

► *Install extra locks* on your exterior doors, sliding glass doors, and windows, and *use* them. All exterior doors should be equipped with a 1-inch deadbolt, including a security strike plate with 3-inch screws.

► *Install a 180-degree door viewer.* A one-way peephole is inexpensive and easily installed. Check at your hardware store when you buy one to see if someone from the store is available to install it.

► *Check out visitors.* The peephole will allow you to see anyone who knocks on your door. *Always* inspect their photo ID before opening the door and letting them into your home. Look outside for a service truck, and notice whether they are wearing an appropriate uniform. Identification can be forged. If you have any reason to doubt the person at your door, call the service company to verify who they are. Never let a stranger into your home.

► *Don't open the door,* if you still feel uncomfortable. Ask the caller to return in 30 minutes or an hour. This will give you time to contact a friend or relative, who can come over and be there when the caller returns.

► *Check vendor licenses.* Vendors in cities are required to obtain licenses and should be able to present them on request. Don't conduct business with anyone selling door to door who doesn't have one; but remember that a license doesn't guarantee the quality of work that the company does.

▶ *Ask for ID.* If the person at the door refuses to show identification and will not leave, excuse yourself for a moment and say you'll be right back. Then notify the police. Telephone your doorman or building superintendent if you live in an apartment.

▶ *Add exterior lights that come on when someone approaches.* They will light your doorways, and they will also startle intruders and make them visible to you and your neighbors.

▶ *Don't hide your keys outside the house.* Instead, leave an extra set with someone you trust, perhaps a neighbor, friend, or relative. Be sure to give them the code to your alarm, if you have one.

▶ *Tell your neighbors about any changes in your schedule* or anyone you expect to visit, such as delivery men, repairmen, and friends or family. This way, they will notice anyone who is a stranger, and, at the same time, they will be keeping an eye on your property. Be sure to exchange the favor. You will develop a relationship with someone on whom you can depend in an emergency, and it's a good way to get to know others who are close by.

▶ *Be sure your street address number is large, freshly painted or well lit, and unobstructed,* so police and emergency personnel can find your home quickly.

▶ *"Wander-proof" your home,* if necessary. Install alarms and hang bells on doors, so that you are alerted to night movement by possible intruders. These are also effective tools for residents who struggle with dementia or Alzheimer's disease, and might wander at night.

▶ *Use only your first initial in phone books, directories, and apartment lobbies.* If you live alone, minimize the number of people who know about it.

▶ *Hang up immediately on obscene or harassing phone calls.* If the caller persists, call the phone company and the police.

▶ *Don't keep large sums of money in your home.*

▶ *Don't give out house or car keys,* credit cards, checkbooks, or savings account passbooks to a housekeeper, home health worker, or caregiver.

▶ *Use a safe deposit box.* Keep stock certificates, bonds, seldom-worn or very expensive jewelry, and stamp and coin collections in a safe deposit box.

▶ *Use direct deposit* for Social Security or pension checks.

## HOME MODIFICATIONS FOR ELDERLY VISITORS

Although modifications to your home depend on your visitor's needs, some simple changes will create a safer environment and prevent falls. Falls are particularly dangerous for the elderly because their skin is thinner and more susceptible to cuts and bruises, and breaks are common because their bones are fragile.

▶ *Remove scatter rugs.* A toe, cane, or walker could easily catch and cause a trip or fall.

▶ *Brighten your lighting* to reduce the risk of falls, cuts, and burns. Use at least 60-watt bulbs in most rooms, and at least 100-watt bulbs for reading.

▶ *Place night-lights throughout key pathways in your home,* for example, along the route to the bathroom.

▶ *Remove all clutter in the house.*

▶ *Allow lots of space for stopping and sitting.*

▶ *Make stairways and steps stand out.* Use brightly colored electrical tape to mark the edge of each step, both in the house and outside.

▶ *Improve lighting for stairways.* Sunlight can cause glare, making it more difficult to see the steps. If there is a window at the top or bottom of a staircase, put up a window shade and make the overhead lighting brighter.

▶ *Move electrical cords out of the way.* Older adults with low vision may have trouble seeing them. If you must extend a cord across an area where your visitor will walk, use tape to secure it to the floor and call attention to it. *Don't* cover the cord with a rug—it just makes it easier to trip over.

▶ *Move lamps and other appliances closer to the walls,* so that electrical cords don't extend into traffic areas.

▶ *Rearrange your furniture.* Move low furniture, such as coffee tables, out of high-traffic areas. Create pathways for walkers or wheelchairs.

▶ *Move chairs closer together.* This can make conversation easier if your visitor has difficulty hearing.

▶ *Inspect your seating.* Getting out of a soft-cushioned or low chair can prove challenging. Adjust your cushions and put a board underneath the seat if it's really soft. Raise the height of a chair by placing a pillow or folded blanket on the seat.

▶ *Lower the water temperature.* Most hot water heaters are set at 150°F—hot enough to scald within seconds. If you have access to your water heater, turn the temperature down to 110°F, or the low setting. If you can't adjust your water heater, consider faucets and valves that prevent scalding. You can buy one specifically to prevent a change in water temperature if someone flushes the toilet.

▶ *Use a bathmat or textured strip on the floor* outside the tub or shower to prevent slipping on a wet floor. Apply non-slip mats and strips to the floor of your bathtub or shower to reduce the risk of falls while bathing.

▶ *Move bedroom lamps closer to the bed.* Lamps and lighting in the bedroom should be easily reached from the bed. That way your visitors won't need to walk from the light switch to the bed in the dark.

## FIRE SAFETY

Americans over the age of 65 have a death rate from fire that is nearly twice the national average. For those over 75, this jumps to three times the national average, and the number of incidents quadruples after age 85.

These statistics are especially alarming because researchers estimate that, by 2030, the 65-and-older population will exceed 70 million people.

Senior citizens are at greater risk of dying in a fire than the rest of the population because their thinner skin is more vulnerable, their reflexes are slower, and they're more likely to be taking medication that makes them drowsy. A particularly deadly combination occurs if the older person combines medication with alcohol or smoking.

According to the United States Fire Administration, adults 65 years and older can reduce this death rate by changing six major fire safety habits:

1. *Install a fire alarm and change the batteries regularly.* The National Fire Protection Association reports that residential fire deaths have dramatically decreased because people have installed more smoke detectors.

   You can more than double your chances of surviving a fire by having a working smoke alarm. Make sure alarms are installed on each level of your home and outside all sleeping areas. If you sleep with the bedroom doors closed, a smoke alarm should be installed in each room. If you or a parent lives in a high-rise building or care facility, check with the building manager to be sure enough smoke detectors are available for the space.

   If your alarms are more than 10 years old—either battery-operated or wired into the building's electrical system—the components aren't reliable and should be replaced. Test each alarm monthly and replace the battery at least once a year.

   Adults who are deaf or hard of hearing should invest in visual aids, such as alarms with blinking lights. Flashing or vibrating smoke alarms should also be tested every month. Vacuum the outside of the smoke detector, because dust impairs effectiveness.

2. *Create new escape routes.* Many older adults are still using escape routes that were planned when their children were living in the house—and when they were significantly younger and more agile.

Create a new plan to escape fire that includes *two* ways to get out of each room, and then *practice it*. Consider your capabilities when preparing escape routes. Make sure all exits are accessible for walkers or wheelchairs, if necessary.

It's a good idea to keep a pair of slippers, eyeglasses, and a flashlight next to your bed, so that, if you hear your smoke alarm at night, you will be prepared to get out of your home quickly. Once you hear the alarm, every second counts.

Don't worry about your pets. They are usually able to get out on their own, and there is no time to gather them or your belongings. Noxious fumes could overcome you at any moment, so don't delay.

During a fire, the cleanest air is 12 inches above the floor, so practice crawling to the nearest safe exit. If you can, cover your mouth and nose with a wet handkerchief or washcloth to filter out the smoke.

If you're in a strange building, memorize the number of doors from your door to a lighted stairwell—doors can be counted if it's too dark to see. Touch all doors first before opening them. If the door or the doorknob is hot to the touch, you can be sure fire is burning on the other side and you *should not open that particular door*.

Never use elevators in a fire emergency. Everyone must use the stairwells to leave the building. If you are unable to use stairs, find the safest place to wait for help. Look for a space that has a door to keep the smoke out, a phone to call 911 for help, and windows from which to signal.

Put on your glasses, grab your flashlight and cell phone, and take a washcloth with you to wave or cover your mouth. If there is a balcony, wait outside and be sure you have gotten someone's attention.

If you are cognitively impaired or disabled physically and cannot move quickly, sleep on the ground floor. Install a fire alarm and a carbon monoxide detector in your room. If you have trouble hearing, buy a special-needs alarm that flashes or has a louder sound.

3. *Plan your escape before there is a fire.* Call the fire department for suggestions about how to deal with your specific challenge, and then implement them. If others live in the house, assign someone specifically to help you get out. Practice what you will do with your partner. If necessary, alter doors to accommodate wheelchairs and add ramps, if needed.

   If a fire occurs, call 911 to report it, even if someone else has already called. Let them know where you are, that you are trapped, and whether you have any disability. If you use a teletypewriter or a telecommunications device for the deaf, keep it next to your bed.

   Close as many doors between you and the fire as possible. If you can, seal vents with duct tape or wet cloths, and put a wet towel along the bottom of the door. This will minimize smoke until help arrives. Wait by the window and signal the fireman with a flashlight or a light colored cloth. Keep a cell or cordless phone with you at all times.

4. *Change unsafe smoking habits.* Careless smoking is the leading cause of fire deaths among people 65 years and older. Make sure you stay alert when you smoke. When you are finished smoking, soak the ashes in water before discarding them. Never leave smoking materials unattended. Use deep ashtrays.

   Smokers should never smoke in bed. They shouldn't smoke when tired or around flammable objects. They should check furniture for embers that can smolder for hours before bursting into flame.

5. *Practice safety in the kitchen to prevent fires.* Cooking fires are the leading cause of fire injuries among older adults. When using the stove, never leave cooking food unattended. Turn off the stove if you need to step away.

Don't leave the kitchen while you are cooking. If you have to leave the kitchen to answer the doorbell or talk on the phone, set a timer or take a spoon to remind yourself that you are cooking.

Wear close-fitting clothing when cooking over an open flame; a dangling sleeve can catch fire easily. Keep towels and potholders away from the flame.

6. *Use safe heating practices.* Maintain heating equipment. Have it checked and serviced by a licensed heating and air conditioning company.

Do not store newspapers, rags, or other combustible materials near a furnace, hot water heater, or space heater. Keep flammable materials, such as curtains or furniture, at least 3 feet from space heaters. Never use a stove as a substitute for a furnace or space heater.

For more information on senior fire safety or other fire safety topics, write to the United States Fire Administration, Public Fire Education, Building I, 16825 South Seton Avenue, Emmitsburg, MD 21727, or visit http://www.usfa.fema.gov.

# Safety on the Road

*To Drive or Not to Drive?*

*Dear Ageless:*

Sometimes, my 72-year-old father is a perfectly competent driver. Other times, he's an accident about to happen. I'm worried and confused about what to do for him and what I can do to anticipate this problem in my own life.

*Sad for Dad*

*Dear Sad for Dad:*

The National Highway Traffic Safety Administration has reported that drivers older than 70 are involved in more crashes per mile than any other age group. Many older drivers react too slowly in emergency situations, causing 14 percent of all traffic fatalities and 18 percent of all pedestrian deaths each year. Seniors who have lost their ability to drive safely put themselves and others on the road in danger. They are more likely to have multiple accidents, and a person 65 or older who is involved in a car accident is more likely to be seriously hurt, more likely to be hospitalized, and more likely to die than younger people involved in the same crash.

*Degenerating vision, poor hearing, and drowsiness caused by medication are generally the causes. Call the American Association of Retired People at 888-227-7669, or visit www.AARP.org, for the list of warning signs for when someone should limit or stop driving. Also, visit www.seniordrivers.org for resource links and more information about how to handle this sensitive and life-altering situation.*

*Ageless*

Losing the option to drive affects a person in many ways—logistically, physically, and psychologically. It signifies the loss of freedom, independence, and self-sufficiency; it can affect the ability to hold a job; and it can reduce involvement in social and community activities. It's such a significant loss that most people resist giving up their license for as long as possible, and often drive far longer than they should.

Even if the senior agrees that a problem exists, resistance to making the final decision can take many forms, including depression, sadness, and anger. It's critical to handle this problem carefully, methodically, and with compassion.

Begin by taking the senior to a physician to determine whether medications being taken or a physical impairment might be the problem. Suggest that it might be as simple as changing a prescription or improving the ability to see or hear. Perhaps new glasses, a hearing aid, or cataract removal might be all that is needed to improve the ability to drive.

## MEDICATIONS AND DRIVING

Driving when you're drowsy is the leading cause of crashes, and it is just as dangerous as drunk driving. Nearly 20 percent of seniors drive under the influence of medication that can make them sleepy. A physician should determine whether the medications being taken (including over-the-counter drugs) and any drug combinations are safe, and whether they can affect judgment or reaction time. The driver also should be examined for chronic diseases, such as muscle atrophy, osteoporosis, or arthritis that might impact strength and flexibility.

After beginning any new medication, seniors should wait four days before driving again. Adverse side effects, including drowsiness, are worse at the start of medication use. The senior should also avoid driving in the middle of the afternoon if they are accustomed to taking a nap then, or late at night when they are usually in bed.

## Is Vision a Problem?

Aging affects peripheral vision, light sensitivity, and the ability to focus quickly. A 60-year-old driver needs three times as much light to see as a teenager, and takes twice as long to adjust to changes in light. See an ophthalmologist for a thorough eye exam.

Everyone over age 50 should have a comprehensive annual exam by an ophthalmologist, who will test for many conditions, including near- and farsightedness, high pressure in the eyes that can cause glaucoma (a leading cause of blindness), and harmful changes that can result from diabetes.

At the same time, she will make sure that the prescription for your glasses and/or contact lenses is correct. Call EyeCare America at 800-222-3937 to see if you qualify for a free exam and treatment.

*Presbyopia*, or "farsightedness," is the impairment of vision most associated with aging. It results from a change in the ratio of water to protein in the eye lens, which makes the lens less flexible and able to focus. Additionally, the crystalline lens of the eye loses elasticity, causing the point of clear vision to be farther away.

Numerous conditions can cause a loss in visual clarity, including cataracts and dry eye, which is sometimes the result of dehydration or medications for lowering cholesterol and combating allergies. Both problems must be corrected for health, comfort, and improved eyesight.

*Presbyopia, or "far-sightedness," is the impairment of vision most associated with aging. It results from a change in the ratio of water to protein in the eye lens, which makes the lens less flexible and able to focus. Additionally, the crystalline lens of the eye loses elasticity, causing the point of clear vision to be farther away.*

A healthy lifestyle beginning in our 20s can help prevent cataracts and macular degeneration of the retina. Give up smoking, drink in moderation, and avoid ultraviolet (UV) light by always wearing sunglasses outside.

Eat a diet rich in vitamins C and E, beta-carotene, and the nutrients lutein and zeaxanthin, which are found in eggs, kale, spinach, turnip and collard greens, romaine lettuce, broccoli, zucchini, peas, and Brussels sprouts. If you don't eat five servings of fruits and vegetables a day, consider a multivitamin/multi-mineral supplement that includes components specific to eye health.

Investigate the available vision correction procedures to see if this might be helpful. The main ones are cataract surgery, usually accompanied by the implantation of an intraocular lens to provide good vision at all distances, and LASIK, a refractory laser eye surgery that reshapes the cornea and can correct near- or farsightedness as well as astigmatism.

Be sure to read the layman-friendly book *Mayo Clinic on Vision and Eye Health: Practical Answers on Glaucoma, Cataracts, Macular Degeneration & Other Conditions* by Helmut Buettner and, in addition to getting an annual eye exam, check that the brightness on the instrument panel of the car is on high, and clean the windshield, mirrors, and headlights.

## HEARING ISSUES

Reacting appropriately is impossible if a driver is unable to hear horns, screeching tires, or sirens. Have your hearing tested by an audiologist and, if necessary, consider getting hearing aids, which are now smaller, more comfortable, and highly sensitive. Try various types before making a purchase.

If it is necessary to correct hearing with an aid, *be sure to wear it*, and make sure that it is functioning properly. Adjusting a hearing aid can be very difficult, so choose a type that can be operated easily.

## ANALYZE DRIVING ABILITY

Everyone ages differently, so some people are perfectly capable of continuing to drive in their 70s, 80s, and even beyond. However, many older people are at higher risk for accidents. If you or another older driver is experiencing trouble on the road, it's important to monitor the situation carefully. Here are some signs to watch for:

- ▶ Changes in general behavior and health
- ▶ Range-of-motion problems—difficulty looking over the shoulder or moving arms, hands, and feet
- ▶ Trouble moving the foot from the gas to the brake pedal, or confusing the two pedals
- ▶ Feeling more nervous or fearful while driving, or feeling exhausted after driving
- ▶ Not understanding why others are honking
- ▶ Getting frustrated while driving
- ▶ Reluctance or refusal from others to be in the car when the senior is driving
- ▶ Increased number of traffic tickets
- ▶ Drifting into other lanes
- ▶ Driving on the wrong side of the road or the shoulder
- ▶ Abrupt lane changes
- ▶ Braking or accelerating too quickly or too slowly
- ▶ Slow reaction to changes in driving conditions

▶ Driving too slowly for existing traffic conditions and speed limits

▶ Almost crashing or more frequent close calls

▶ Dents and scrapes on the car, garage doors, mailboxes, or fences

▶ Failing to use the turn signal or failing to turn it off

▶ Keeping turn signals on without changing lanes

▶ Difficulty following directions

▶ Getting lost more often, especially in familiar locations

▶ Not paying attention to signals, signs, or pedestrians

## SAFE DRIVING TIPS FOR DRIVERS WHO ARE BEGINNING TO HAVE PROBLEMS

▶ *Consider special equipment.* Have an occupational therapist determine whether special equipment will optimize reaction time and make it easier to operate a car.

▶ *Avoid driving in bad weather.*

▶ *Drive only during daylight hours* if you have trouble seeing well in reduced light.

▶ *Plan your route before you leave the house.* Check Mapquest, Google Maps, and Yahoo Maps for directions. Consider buying a global positioning system (GPS).

▶ *Stay off highways if you are bothered by fast moving traffic.* Mapquest has an "avoid highways" routing alternative under "*Advanced Options.*"

▶ *Carry a cell phone* for emergencies, but don't use it while driving.

▶ *Keep hands on the wheel.* Don't adjust controls, position mirrors, or change radio stations while driving. Some cars have controls for the radio on the steering wheel that require no reaching and no looking away from the road.

▶ *Don't eat, drink, or converse while driving,* to avoid being distracted.

▶ *Yield to the other driver,* if you're not sure who has the right of way.

▶ *Use the 3-second rule* to determine how closely to follow the car ahead of you. Choose a stationary object on the road ahead, start counting when the car in front of you passes the object, and then allow 3 seconds until you pass the object. You can figure 3 seconds by saying to yourself, "a thousand one, a thousand two, a thousand three." If you pass the chosen object in less than 3 seconds, maintain a longer following distance.

▶ *Move to the right.* If you would rather drive slowly, move into the right lane or pull over and allow other cars to pass you.

▶ *Enroll in a driver safety course for people over 50.* Visit www.aarp.org/families/driver_safety, or call 1-888-227-7669, to find a course in your area. The refresher course takes 8 hours and costs just $10. Check with your insurance company about a reduction in the cost of your premium after you complete the course.

## THE DIFFICULT CONVERSATION

If a resolution to problems with driving is not possible, you may have to insist that a senior stop driving. This is a very serious discussion that will require prior thought and careful treading. The American Association of Retired People (AARP) makes the following suggestions for how to handle this delicate situation:

▶ *Be understanding* about resistance, anger, and even depression. This is a terrible milestone to face.

▶ *Ask questions* rather than make demands.

▶ *Discuss safety issues* and your fear that the senior will hurt himself or others.

▶ *Point out any tickets or accidents* as part of the reason for your concern.

▶ *Seek confirmation* from the driver about the situation. Some older drivers know it's time to stop driving, but they aren't sure how they will handle life without being able to drive. They may even feel relieved to have someone else help them make the decision to stop driving.

▶ *Be prepared with options.*

▶ *Offer to gives rides and run errands.*

▶ *Be available.* If you're able to, say you will be there on a regular basis to do chores such as going to the grocery store.

According to a survey conducted by The Hartford Insurance Company, many older adults think that family members should talk with them when potential problems arise. In their study, 50 percent of older adults said that having a serious accident is an opportunity to start a conversation, and 33 percent said a minor accident or narrowly avoiding an accident should also trigger a conversation.

For more information, visit www.thehartford.com/talkwitholder drivers/having/conversopeners.htm for more information.

The following situations provide opportunities to talk about driving skills:

▶ Health changes

▶ Self-regulation of driving

▶ Car accidents

▶ Near misses

## QUESTIONS TO START A DIALOGUE

The Hartford Insurance Company website suggests starting the discussion with questions that don't sensationalize difficult circumstances. For example, try saying or asking:

▶ *"I'm glad you've cut down on night driving. I appreciate your not driving when you're uncomfortable or feel that it's too risky."* When adults modify their driving in small ways without guidance from others, families should praise self-regulation as a positive step and not discourage the driver's actions. For example, don't dismiss the older adult as a worrier, or discourage a driver who is limiting night driving by leaving a family event before dark. Be supportive, and express your willingness to support their transportation needs.

▶ *"Have you asked your doctor about the effects of your new medication on your driving?"* Many medications have sedative effects that can prevent a person from processing information quickly. About 75 percent of older adults think a significant change in their health is a legitimate reason to have a discussion about driving.

▶ *"That was a close call yesterday. I'm worried about your safety on the road."* In situations where the older driver was not at fault, families might want to discuss the driver's diminishing ability to drive defensively. This type of discussion is always more productive if it is not held at the scene of an accident.

▶ *"I'm worried you might get lost."* Almost 70 percent of older adults say that getting lost while driving is a valid reason to discuss their ability to drive. Getting lost in a familiar place may suggest potentially serious cognitive health issues that could affect driving skills. This might also be a good time to get a doctor involved in the discussion.

## WHAT TO DO IF HIGH-RISK DRIVERS REFUSE TO STOP DRIVING

Additional information from the Hartford Insurance Company may help with difficult situations. According to the company's informative website: "Some older drivers will not respond to even the most logical and constructive conversations. In that case, you will have to take drastic measures. Remember, you are protecting her from harming herself and others. You might have to:

▶ Disable the car

▶ Take away the car

▶ Remove the keys from the senior's possession

▶ Cancel the vehicle registration

▶ Prevent the older driver from renewing his driver's license

▶ Speak with the driver's doctor about the problem; solicit his support

▶ Schedule a formal driving assessment

To learn about state motor vehicle driver testing, call your state licensing agency or consult the Insurance Institute for Highway Safety at www.iihs.org. Be aware that the driver you are attempting to protect may counteract your measures. Solicit as much 'legal' support as possible, and as much evidence. With patience, you can ultimately convince the driver that this is the best solution for everyone."

## HELPING SENIORS HANDLE THE SITUATION

Losing your driver's license is life-changing—it will affect the driver and anyone living in the same household. It's imperative to make the transition as smooth as possible. Consider the following:

▶ *Discuss the situation.* The process will be easier if you include the senior in the discussion as much as possible.

▶ *Allow the person to keep as much control as possible;* this is extremely important in maintaining dignity and self-respect.

▶ *Let them keep the car.* If an elderly driver can keep her own car, she may adjust better to not driving it. If a spouse or others can drive her in her own car, it will make the situation easier to handle.

▶ *Research all possible forms of transportation in the area*—routes, schedules, and costs. Provide a one-page list of contact numbers, including taxi services.

▶ *Check into home delivery* and show the senior how to use the Internet to make purchases. Collect various catalogs for him. Help him place orders until he learns how to do it himself.

▶ *Continuity is critical* if the elderly driver is to believe that the change will be tolerable. Make sure nothing disrupts her schedule—which should be developed together. Put all appointments on a calendar for her—and you. Include social and church activities, and arrange for her to get to all of them.

▶ *Make being home as enjoyable as possible.* If the house needs attention, take care of it. Make the environment lovely and neat, and be sure that the refrigerator and pantry are always well stocked.

▶ *Encourage hobbies*—old and new—reading, games, puzzles, and crafts to do while at home and on car trips. Participate, at least at first, until new skills are integrated.

▶ *Encourage an upbeat attitude.* Help her to feel positive about changes in her environment. Be sure to compliment all progress. Be affirming.

▶ *Anticipate the senior's needs, and make sure you offer to help*—and that others do, too. Asking for rides is one of the most difficult parts of not driving.

## Ensure Continuing Mobility

▶ *Contact senior-service organizations for help.* Call the Eldercare Locator for options.

▶ *Use your local Area Agency on Aging* to direct you to available programs.

▶ *Check out the AARP's state-by-state transportation options list.*

▶ *Contact the American Public Transportation Association.*

▶ *Contact the Red Cross and American Cancer Society.* These organizations have a variety of programs, including transporting people in need.

▶ *Ask about congregation-based rides.* Interfaith and church-based programs include transporting others.

▶ *Arrange car pools* or sharing rides with friends and relatives.

▶ *Accompany the person on public transportation*—buses, subways, and light rail—until he is comfortable to ride alone.

▶ *Arrange for taxis, limousines, chauffeur services,* and private drivers, if necessary.

▶ *Investigate transit that is intended specifically for seniors.*

▶ *Suggest a bicycle;* consider a three-wheeler made especially for older and handicapped riders.

▶ *Encourage walking*—he will get exercise, too.

▶ *Buy a motorized wheelchair* for non-ambulatory seniors.

▶ *Consider an adult day care center* as a way to get seniors out and socializing. Transportation is generally included.

Most people believe that having a car and a driver's license are critical to their independence and ability to be self-sufficient, and losing the right to drive can be extremely upsetting. However, for obvious reasons, compromised drivers must not be allowed to drive. If this situation arises—with a little preparation and a lot of sensitivity—most seniors can be persuaded to give up driving for their own safety and the safety of others.

# Avoiding Scams and Fraud

## *Refuse to Be a Victim*

*Dear Ageless:*

*My mother was really "taken" by a con artist. Her roof had been pummeled by hail and was leaking badly. Because so many homes had been damaged in the storm, most of the well-known companies in the area were backlogged. When a man stopped by and said he could fix it for her in just a couple of days with material that would last a lifetime, she invited him in. He was a real sweet-talker and convinced her to pay half up front to buy the materials. He assured her that if the job was in any way unsatisfactory, she would not have to pay the other half, although he was entirely sure she would be more than satisfied with the job they would do.*

*Needless to say, her check was cashed immediately, and he and "his crew" disappeared. What can I do to protect her and the rest of my family members from these loathsome scoundrels?*

*Sincerely Disgusted*

*Dear Sincerely Disgusted:*

*Senior citizens are often approached by individuals offering to perform various home repair jobs such as fixing roofs,* driveways, gutters and asphalt, trimming trees, and painting exteriors. The perpetrators claim to have materials left over from other jobs, offer significant discounts, or even say that a close relative or friend sent them.

Many complete the job, but the cost of the work is suddenly more than the first quote, and payment in cash is demanded. The con artists may even offer to provide a ride to the bank, so that the victim can convert her check into cash. Other times, like in your mom's case, the crook just cashes in the "earnest money" and disappears.

Con artists are good at what they do; they have no conscience about duping people, and no conscience about stealing from people on fixed incomes who can least afford it. They do not prey only on senior citizens, however. They are equal opportunity criminals, and anyone can be a target.

You must take charge of your life. Be alert in your home, on the telephone, and in your community. Assume that if it sounds too good to be true, it is, and if you don't know the person who is trying to sell you something, proceed with caution. It's always best to work with people whose services have been used by a family member or friend, preferably more than once.

Ageless

As we grow older and gain experience, we become more afraid of being the victim of a crime. For many people who have been victimized, the trauma changes their outlook about their community. They become fearful and feel that their security and the quality of their lives have been jeopardized—and, indeed, they have been adversely impacted. The fear is sometimes so debilitating that they begin locking themselves in their homes. This results in isolation, which is one of the main causes of the vulnerability that these criminals depend on. It's truly a vicious cycle.

Statistics suggest, however, that a person is *less likely* to be a victim of a violent crime as they grow older, so jailing ourselves in our homes is not necessary or advisable. We must refuse to allow criminals to steal our freedom as well as our assets.

The reality is that seniors are most often the target of pickpockets, purse snatchers, and con artists. These people have developed intricate frauds and con games targeted specifically at senior citizens.

To avoid being victimized, be on the alert for some of these, the most common scams and problems perpetrated on older people and those who care for them.

## HOME REPAIRS

When hiring a worker for any job, it's critical to take the time to check their references. However, be wary of even these, because you really have no idea whose names and numbers they've given you. The references could all be their relatives or other members of their gang. Often these crooks run in packs, moving from one area to another, preying on the vulnerable.

Always check with the Better Business Bureau. If the company is not listed with them, do not use their services. If the company is listed, check to see if any complaints have been lodged against them. Call the national office of the Council of Better Business Bureaus at 1-703-276-0100, or visit www.us.bbb.org. Enter your zip code at www.bbb.org, to locate your local bureau for information about companies and charities.

You can also contact your County Clerk's Office to see if any complaints have been registered there against the company.

Do not pay for a job until it's done, and then only after you or another professional has inspected the quality of the work. If you believe that the contractor is not doing a good job, or you feel threatened in any way, contact your local police and your attorney prior to making payment.

## DIVERSION BURGLARIES

This scam has several variations. One type usually occurs during the spring, summer, or fall, when people are working outside and rarely lock the doors to their homes. One of the thieves approaches the victim and gets his attention, while the second thief enters the victim's home and steals cash, jewelry, silver, and whatever else can be easily collected and carried away.

Another diversion technique can happen any time. The thieves come to the front door and ask for a drink of water, to use a bathroom or a telephone, or for help with an emergency. While one thief has the victim's attention, the accomplice searches for valuables.

Be careful, even if a woman comes to your door. We have a tendency to be more trusting of women. If a woman is part of a group of criminals, however, she may be the face you see in the peephole while the men stand out of view.

Do the following, regardless of who comes knocking:

▶ *Don't let strangers in.* If an unknown person comes to your home seeking directions, the phone, the bathroom, or other assistance, keep them outside your home and have at least one locked door between you and them.

  − If they ask for water, direct them to an outside faucet.
  − If they say they need to contact someone, offer to make the call for them.

▶ *Keep doors locked.* When working in the yard, leave only one door unlocked that you can visibly monitor at all times.

▶ *Install an alarm system,* if you can afford it. Thieves who are deterred by alarm systems will leave when they read the exterior sign and the labels on your windows saying that you have one.

▶ *Get a dog.* Barking dogs are a good deterrent, particularly a *big* barking dog.

## BANK EXAMINER SCAM

In this scenario, the con artist poses as a bank official, police officer, or FBI agent. He flashes a badge or other identification (which can be easily faked), and suggests that a problem has occurred with the victim's bank account. He asks the victim to help him "catch" the bank employee suspected of fraud. The plan includes the victim withdrawing and turning over large sums of money to be used in the "sting." Of course, neither the money nor the official is ever seen again.

Professionals, such as bank officials and police officers, have other ways of conducting criminal investigations that do not involve innocent people. They have their own undercover officers and money for covert operations to check for bank fraud.

If you are approached by this type of con artist, contact their claimed employer (in the example given above, this would be the bank) to verify their employment. If the person claims to be a detective or FBI agent, ask for a uniformed officer to come to your location to verify their identity. Check all identification carefully. If you suspect that something is wrong, excuse yourself and call 911.

## LETTER SCAM

The swindler in this scheme claims to be from a foreign country (usually in the developing world) and that he has inherited a large sum of money. He produces a letter stating that—under the law in his country—he cannot return to his country with more than a small amount of U.S. currency.

The swindler asks for the victim's help. The suggested plan is for the victim to keep the money and periodically send small amounts back to him in his home country.

The con artist tells his victim that he trusts him, but that it will be necessary for the victim to prove she has money of her own, so that she won't be tempted to keep any of the con artist's money.

When the victim withdraws a large sum of money from her bank, the money is placed into a handkerchief or envelope along with the con artist's money, and a switch is made. The victim is later given an identical envelope or handkerchief containing cut-up paper, and the con artist disappears.

Variations on this scam can also show up as e-mails from people in foreign countries claiming to need your help with an inheritance. Just delete them.

## INVESTMENT SCAMS

Con artists are usually clean-cut, well dressed, and personable. They do not look like crooks or in any way disreputable. They are talented sales people who are in the business of getting you to give them your money.

Be very careful if someone encourages you to invest in a get-rich quick scheme. Follow these tips when considering a financial investment:

▶ *Buy only from licensed financial professionals.* They are trained and certified.

▶ *Regularly review your account statements.* This is your money. No one will care about it like you do.

▶ *Buy investment products only after you have researched them carefully.*

▶ *Make sure all your investments are registered with the Securities Exchange Commission (SEC).*

▶ *Ignore spam e-mail* and all "hot tips" when it comes to investing.

▶ *Be careful if you're invited to participate in a scheme at a social event.* Take time to research any proposal.

▶ *Never buy into a "sure thing."* Nothing is guaranteed; all investments carry a risk.

▶ *Never pay an individual,* if you do decide to invest. The check should be made out to the financial institution he represents.

▶ *Get the facts.* If your salesperson—and that's what brokers really are, because most represent certain products for which they get a commission—refuses to answer questions, won't allow you to withdraw your money, or won't provide proper statements, report her to the authorities and the SEC. Visit www.sec.gov for more information.

*Con artists are usually clean-cut, well dressed, and personable. They do not look like crooks or in any way disreputable. They are talented sales people who are in the business of getting you to give them your money.*

## INTERNET SCAMS

Multiple scams float around online, most of which appeal to our desire to earn money. One such scam has to do with "home businesses." The scammers sell you "kits," or over-the-telephone training programs that promise huge profits. The victim pays a great deal of money for a product that has no real value, and for a business that does not generate "thousands of dollars per month."

Another common Internet scam is notification of winning a monetary prize. The requirement for receiving the award, however, is to pay various fees first, and many victims have traveled as far as Europe to do so. Some victims have lost as much as $50,000 in this type of scheme.

If you have any doubt—and you should—about any "prize" won on the Internet, do *not* respond to the e-mail. Instead, contact the local office of the FBI or the National Consumers League at 800-355-9625. They have a list of all the current schemes. Additionally, you might be letting them know about a new scheme that they can warn others about. You could be saving yourself and others a great deal of heartache.

## IDENTITY THEFT

Someone's identity is stolen every 2 seconds. This is staggering and scary. People have lost thousands (sometimes hundreds of thousands) of dollars, not just in the theft itself, but in their attempt to recover their good name and credit, a process that often takes years. You must be vigilant in protecting your personal information. Keep these recommendations handy, so you can quickly review how to handle various situations:

- ▶ *Use a U.S. Post Office or mail store mailbox,* particularly for envelopes that contain checks. Thieves steal mail from curbside mailboxes, wash the checks, rewrite them, and drain your bank accounts. You also risk thieves obtaining important information from your mail that can contribute to identity theft.

- ▶ *Use initials only.* The next time you order checks, have only the initial of your first name and middle name printed with your full last name. If someone steals your checkbook, he will not know if you sign your checks with just your initials or your first name. Your bank will know how you sign your checks and, although tellers do not always check, it might identify the problem sooner. It will also help you prove your case later, if the need arises.

- ▶ *Do not put your complete account number on checks* you write to credit card companies. If you want to put something on the "For" line of your check, put only the last four numbers. The credit card company knows the rest of the number, and anyone who might be handling your check won't have access to it. This is important because checks pass through many processing channels.

- ▶ *Never give your Social Security card number to anyone,* even if they call and say they represent what sounds like a legitimate institution. Tell them you will call the institution with the needed information. Do not call back any number the caller gives you. It will likely be as bogus as the rest of their story.

- ▶ *Put your work telephone number on your checks instead of your home phone.* If you have a post office box number, use that instead of your home address.

▶ *Never have your Social Security number printed on your checks.* You can add it later, if necessary. But if you have it printed, anyone can get it.

▶ *Carry a photocopy of your passport*—in addition to your original passport—in case the original is lost or stolen.

▶ *Copy important documents.* Place the contents of your wallet on a photocopy machine and copy both sides of each license, bank ATM card, and credit card. If your wallet is stolen, you will know what you had in it, as well as all the account numbers you will need to cancel and the phone numbers that you will need to call. Keep the photocopy in a safe place that you feel burglers won't think of, and/or leave a copy with a friend or family member.

▶ *Do not carry your checkbook* in your purse, unless you need it to make a purchase while you are out shopping. That way, if your purse is snatched, the thief won't get your checkbook, too.

▶ *File a police report immediately if your wallet is lost or stolen.* File the report in the jurisdiction where the item was stolen. This proves to credit providers that you were diligent, and it's a first step toward opening an investigation.

▶ *Institute a fraud alert.* Call the three national credit-reporting organizations immediately to place a fraud alert on your name and Social Security number. If there is an alert on your account— and the person who stole your credit card tries to use the card— the merchant will know your information was stolen, and they will have to contact you by phone to authorize the purchase. This will alert you to a problem, and a very clear paper trail will exist. The telephone numbers of the three national credit report companies are: Equifax: 1-800-525-6285; Experian (formerly TRW): 1-888-397-3742; and Trans Union: 1-800-680-7289.

▶ *Call the Social Security fraud line.* The Social Security Administration fraud line can be contacted at 1-800-269-0271.

## TELEPHONE FRAUD

▶ *Never give out personal information on the telephone for any reason.* Do not tell anyone your name, address, marital status, Social Security number, or banking information.

▶ *Do not give any details about your credit cards, phone cards, or bank accounts* to phone solicitors, unless you made the initial telephone call.

▶ *Do not talk with strangers on the telephone.* Tell salespeople and survey-takers to remove your number from their lists. They are required by law to do so. If you have not done so, list your home telephone and your cell phone with the Do Not Call registry. Call 1-888-382-1222, or visit www.DONOTCALL.GOV, to register for free. It takes only seconds to register online.

– A legitimate caller will respect your position and agree to an alternate approach, if the caller is legitimate and the representative actually requires the information.

– If you don't want to set up a meeting, ask the caller for the name of the business and telephone number, so that you can return the call. Then, check the number with the information operator or the telephone book.

– A reputable solicitor should identify himself by name, identify the business on whose behalf he is calling, identify the purpose of the call, and identify the telephone number at which the person, company, or organization making the call can be reached.

– If you hear a delay before the caller begins speaking, it usually means that you are being called randomly by a computer. It's definitely not a personalized call, so just hang up.

– If the caller asks: "Who is this?" you should respond: "Who are you calling?" or "To whom do you wish to speak?" Make the caller identify who she is attempting to call. If you do not receive an appropriate response, hang up.

▶ *Don't fall for anything that sounds too good to be true*—a free vacation, sweepstakes prizes, cures for medical ailments and diseases, or high-yield investment schemes. Be suspicious of anyone who offers you something for free or a chance for quick and easy wealth.

▶ *Don't let anyone rush you into signing something*, such as an insurance policy, contract, or sales agreement. Read these documents carefully. Ask someone you trust to read them as well.

▶ *Check to see if the Buyers' Regret Law applies*, if you are sorry you have agreed to a purchase. You have three days within which to change your mind about a purchase, including something as large as a car. These laws vary from state to state.

▶ *Beware of anyone claiming to represent companies, consumer organizations, or government agencies that offer—for a fee—to recover lost money* from fraudulent telemarketers. As a twist on this same theme, con artists sometimes pretend to be officials trying to "catch" a thief with your assistance.

▶ *Never agree to participate in schemes to catch perpetrators of any crime.*

▶ *Say "No" to anyone asking for money over the phone.* Even those who call representing legitimate concerns should be suspect. If you want to donate to the police or firemen, call and ask where donations can be sent, so they won't have to split the donation with the organization calling on their behalf.

▶ *Call to check with the police if you are suspicious.* Don't hesitate to call and check with the police. The FBI also has local offices, and they will give you information on both telephone and Internet schemes.

▶ *Call your police department or your telephone company* and seek their advice about obscene phone calls, night calls from strangers, or frequent wrong number calls. If necessary, change your phone number.

According to the Better Business Bureau and the Federal Trade Commission, you can reduce your risk of becoming a victim of telemarketing fraud by following these tips:

▶ *Be skeptical* about "too good to be true" telephone offers.
▶ *Resist any pressure* to make an immediate decision.
▶ *Ask for written follow-up* materials that explain the offer.
▶ *Agree to pay no more than the price of a postage stamp* when notified about "winning" a sweepstakes. All legitimate sweepstakes must allow a "no purchase necessary" way to play the game and collect the prize.
▶ *Never provide your credit card or checking account numbers* to a caller from an unfamiliar company without first checking out the company with your Better Business Bureau, state consumer protection agency, or state Attorney General.
▶ *Tell companies that you want to be put on their "do not call" list*, to reduce the number of unwanted telephone solicitations you receive.

We have a particular obligation to honor and serve the aging citizens in our society—not just those in our families of origin—but in our human family as well. They must be helped with the activities of daily living, home repairs and maintenance, transportation, and a myriad of other needs. Sometimes the problems are so multifaceted that even caregivers have trouble knowing where to begin.

Answers are readily available. Call 211 and be connected 24 hours a day, 7 days a week to knowledgeable resource and referral specialists who will direct you to a multitude of community services and lots of free information.

The national 211 program was instituted in July, 2000 by the Federal Communications Commission (FCC), and it's funded by federal and state agencies. Visit www.211.org to find a list of 2-1-1 program locations, and to see how services vary from state-to-state.

When you call, it's critical to be detailed in your description of the problems. The 211 specialists will be better able to refer you to the proper providers and agencies, and they may suggest other services for which you are eligible, including assistance with finances, housing, and utilities; medical care and prescriptions; food and transportation; legal needs; childcare; camps; education; employment; and protective services. For a wealth of information, you can also access the 211 database by visiting www.irissoft.com/uwsa.

*Call 211 and be connected 24 hours a day, 7 days a week to knowledgeable resource and referral specialists who will direct you to a multitude of community services and lots of free information.*

By arming yourself with information and taking preventative actions, you can avoid being the victim of a crime—no matter what your age or condition.

# Taking Control

## *Safety Away from Home*

*Dear Ageless:*

*I was recently mugged, and now I'm afraid to go out. I intellectually understand that it is unlikely to happen again, but I feel insecure and vulnerable.*

*Sadly Housebound*

*Dear Housebound:*

*You have every right to feel as you do, and you should take all the time you need to deal with what was certainly a terrible experience. You might want to consider counseling or a support group to help you with the process of reentering the world, because you certainly don't want the criminals to win.*

*The most unscrupulous people in society are the ones who prey on those they believe to be weak. The majority of street crimes are crimes of opportunity. The thief is looking for an easy target: a woman walking down a quiet street, a man carrying bags, or a senior citizen who has just cashed his pension check.*

*It might also be a chance crime—the thief decides that this is the right place and the right time, and you just happen to be* there. Hit-and-run thieves are generally males or teenagers, and they will be strangers.

The most common street crime is purse snatching. The thief catches you unaware, grabs your purse (or cuts the shoulder strap), and runs. Often it happens so quickly that you can't do anything about it, and you cannot identify the person who has robbed you.

Sometimes, men have their wallets taken. This happens less often and usually by force. As long as criminals see an opportunity to take advantage, they will, but you can and should protect yourself.

*Ageless*

## AVOIDING CRIME ON THE STREET

Be particularly careful if crimes are a problem in your neighborhood, and use common sense approaches such as these:

- *Do not carry large sums of money.*
- *Use direct deposit* for any checks you receive regularly, if possible— Social Security, pension payments, and paychecks can all be deposited electronically.
- *Do not flash your money* for others to see.
- *Do not carry valuables* in full view, and only carry what is absolutely necessary.
- *Carry credit cards only when you need them.*
- *Carry your purse close to your body*, preferably in front and not dangling by the straps, which makes it easier for cut-and-run thieves. *Do not* wrap purse straps around your wrist, or you could be dragged along or knocked to the ground in the event of a "snatch."

▶ *Carry a small change purse with only the money or credit cards that you need*, instead of a large handbag with straps. Keep it in your pocket.

▶ *Put your wallet in an inside coat or front pants pocket.*

▶ *Keep all car doors locked at all times.* Be particularly alert for people hanging around in parking lots or garages.

▶ *Park near an entrance or exit of a garage*, if possible. There is more traffic in these areas, and you will have a shorter walk through a dark area.

▶ *Keep packages in the trunk*, not inside the car where others can see them. Thieves will break the windows if the contents of your car are attractive enough.

▶ *Stay alert and tuned into your surroundings.* If someone or something makes you feel uneasy, trust your instincts and leave the area. If necessary, move to where large groups of people are present, even if you don't know them.

▶ *Learn how to use mace or pepper spray* and carry it with you, if you feel comfortable with the idea.

▶ *Go out with family, friends, or a group*, if possible, rather than going alone. Utilize the buddy system—walk in pairs whenever possible.

▶ *Try to walk in a confident, relaxed manner.* Looking afraid makes you appear weak.

▶ *Walk on well-lighted, busy streets.* Stay away from vacant lots, alleys, or construction sites.

▶ *Tell someone where you're going and when you will return.*

▶ *Give up your purse or wallet*, if attacked. Don't risk your personal safety for material loss.

▶ *Consider wearing a whistle*, and blow it if someone is menacing or has attacked you. Someone else may be able to stop them.

▶ *Try to remember the most significant physical characteristic about the offender*, such as a facial scar, a physical deformity, or a distinctive facial characteristic, if you are attacked.

## SAFETY ON PUBLIC TRANSPORTATION

▶ *Pay attention to your surroundings,* and only board and exit public transportation at well-lighted stops.

▶ *Wait near the ticket booth* until you are ready to board a train or subway. Pick a car with several people in it. Don't ride in an empty car.

▶ *Sit near the driver* whenever you ride the bus, trolley, train, or subway.

▶ *Do not fall asleep.* Stay alert.

▶ *Hold on to your packages.*

▶ *Watch who gets on or off with you.* If someone follows you, enter a store or office and call the police. They will take you home.

▶ *Trust your instincts.* If you feel uncomfortable, listen to your misgivings and walk quickly to wherever other people are gathered.

## PARKING LOT SAFETY

The following advice is applicable to anyone, but especially those of us who are growing older and might be viewed by thieves and con artists as more vulnerable, both physically and emotionally. If you are physically fit, you can take these simple steps to protect yourself and learn what actions to take if you are attacked:

▶ *Nothing is worth risking your life.* If someone wants your belongings, don't refuse, but don't just give them over. Toss them as far away as you can, then run in the other direction. If running is not possible, walk as quickly as you can.

▶ *Make yourself a difficult victim.* Before leaving a store, consolidate packages, so they're more manageable. Have your keys in your hand or pocket. Walk purposefully and as quickly as possible to your car.

▶ *Check underneath and inside before opening the car door.* Get in, lock the doors, and leave immediately, so that no one will have time to get in beside you with a weapon.

▶ *Don't drive an intruder anywhere.* If someone is in your car when you get in, don't drive away—even if they have a gun to your head. Floor the engine and drive the car into something. The airbag will protect you. When the car crashes, get out and run. If running is not possible, get out of the car and walk away while yelling for help.

▶ *Refuse to be taken to a second location* (where people have often been tortured, raped, and killed). Instead scream, spray mace, hit the other person's body with your elbows (the strongest point on your body), and kick where you know it will hurt. Be as uncontrollable as you can so that the perpetrator will give up. If you are physically able to do so, consider taking a self-defense class if you feel uncomfortable trying any of these options. You will feel empowered.

▶ *Enter your car from the passenger door* if you're parked next to a big van. Criminals pull women in as they are attempting to get into cars.

▶ *Get the attention of others.* If you're thrown into the trunk, and you are physically able to do so, try to kick out the taillights, stick your arm out of the hole, and wave like crazy. Other drivers will see you and report the car license and description.

▶ *Be careful, paranoid even, but be safe.* If you're uncomfortable in a situation—such as in a dark parking lot or at the mall at night, even at the grocery store—call a security guard or policeman to escort you to your car.

▶ *Carry a cell phone.* They are affordable and easy to use, and they can save your life. Call your provider to see if they have reduced rates for senior citizens. Contact Jitterbug at 1-800-918-8543 to find out about its simple model cell phone, which includes friendly, helpful 24-hour service that can make calls for you, provide directory assistance, and add names to your phone list. The phone has bigger buttons that are backlit and a powerful speaker for people who are having trouble hearing. The cost of the service starts at $10 a month, and there are no long-distance or roaming fees.

Self-empowerment and self-confidence are important at all ages in dealing with potentially dangerous situations. Ready yourself before a situation arises, and don't hesitate to act if necessary.

*Self-empowerment and self-confidence are important at all ages in dealing with potentially dangerous situations. Ready yourself before a situation arises, and don't hesitate to act if necessary.*

Preparation and attitude often dictate outcome. A woman in New York is living proof that taking command of an adverse situation is possible. A robber attempted to steal her purse. Instead of becoming his victim, she smacked him in the head with the purse and caused him to run away. She was 103 years old. That same robber tried and failed to snatch the purse of another elderly lady, because she followed the example of the first woman whose story had made national news. She was 86. Aging doesn't mean we automatically become victims.

# 12

## Depression, Fear, and Grief

### Conquering the Challenges of Aging

Dear Ageless:
My parents are in their late 70s, and they are becoming reclusive. Is this a problem?

Getting Worried

Dear Getting Worried:
According to the Center for Mature Consumer Studies, seniors fall into one of several groups:

"Healthy indulgers: in good health, independent, active, and relatively wealthy, who want to live well and do new things.

Ailing out-goers: in poor health, but socially active and health-conscious. They are concerned about financial matters and security of health, home, and assets.

Healthy hermits: in good health, but have little interest in staying active or making social contacts.

Frail recluses: in poor health, inactive, socially isolated, and psychologically withdrawn. They are concerned about home health care, medical services, and physical security."

If you've noticed your parents changing from one of these categories to another, and you're concerned, discuss it with them. Ask questions about their health. If they haven't seen a physician recently, suggest they make an appointment and go with them. They'll worry less, and you won't be guessing about their well-being.

Don't forget an eye examination. They may not be going out as much because they can't see well enough to drive. You may need to resolve problems of transportation to appointments, shopping, and social activities.

Finances might be an issue. If retirees are living on a fixed income, inflation or insufficient preparation may be taking its toll. Government reports reveal at least one-third of Americans 65 and older have incomes below the poverty level.

Be tactful, but take inventory. Are there dirty clothes and bed linens, an empty refrigerator, or unpaid bills? If they're not able to take care of what are termed activities of daily living (ADLs), you might have to assist with housekeeping or hire outside help.

Loneliness can also be a problem. If they've lost friends or family members, their opportunities for socializing may be dwindling, and methods for engaging in new activities might be unclear. Suggest volunteer work, a part-time job, or joining a group to prevent boredom and lethargy. Visit www.AARP.com for retirement ideas.

Ageless

One of the most challenging aspects of growing older is seeing our parents—and then ourselves—become less capable and independent. It's difficult to watch and then experience our bodies begin to betray us. Physical decline and pain can become constants in our lives, and little else is more debilitating.

Pain can actually change our demeanor—a once positive person can become embittered and angry at this change in circumstance. Pain, if long-lasting or severe enough, can even impact the desire or will to live.

There are two kinds of pain. *Chronic pain* is long-term (lasting more than 6 months). It generally begins with an illness and is controlled with medication. *Acute pain* is short-term, initiated by an illness or injury, managed with narcotics, and alleviated when the injury heals.

Pain is impacted by an individual's physical and mental state, which makes it a unique experience, so even though two people may have the same diagnosis, they may suffer pain differently. Depression, fatigue, and fear make pain harder to bear. Visit the American Academy of Pain Management at www.aapm@aapainmanage.org or call 209-533-9744 for information and a free subscription to their newsletter: *Current Pain Management and Research.*

Pain medication (analgesics), both oral and topical (creams, rubs, and sprays), can give immediate relief. Immobilization, increased circulation (cold, hot, and exercise), sleep, and distraction are effective methods for pain control. Meditation, relaxation, prayer, hypnosis, and deep breathing (increases oxygen to the brain) also alleviate symptoms.

Acupuncture (insertion of needles into acupoints on the body) and acupressure (massage at acupoints) stimulate nerves and release endorphins, and can be effective when administered by those who are well trained, certified, and licensed. Contact the National Certification Commission for Acupuncture and Oriental Medicine (NCCAOM) at www.nccaom.org for referrals.

Transcutaneous (through the skin) nerve stimulators (TNS) send a painless, electrical current to nerves. Generating heat and stimulating the body's production of natural painkillers, the treatment improves mobility, diminishes stiffness, and relieves pain. It's an effective supplement to anti-inflammatory drugs. Biofeedback monitors reactions to conscious and unconscious thoughts by measuring changes in body temperature and blood pressure. Surgery can permanently sever nerves to block pain.

Although pain can be good because it indicates that something is wrong, among seniors, it can become more than transitory, and more than physical in nature. Pain has an emotional component, too—sadness at becoming more fragile and vulnerable, anger at the unfairness of it, and terror about what more can happen. It is no wonder that seniors struggle with fear, grief, and depression.

## DEPRESSION

Depression is a serious medical illness that must be diagnosed and treated by trained professionals. If left untreated, depression can last months or even years, causing unnecessary suffering for the person and his family members.

Depression also makes other diseases worse, leads to disability or premature death, and can result in suicide. People over the age of 65 account for more than 25 percent of the suicides in America.

Being depressed is *not* a normal part of aging, and it's impossible "to just snap out of it." Unlike sadness, which does not affect a person's ability to engage in regular activities, depression interferes with the ability to function.

According to the National Institute of Mental Health, the symptoms of depression include sadness that lasts more than two weeks, unexplained physical pain or gastrointestinal problems, excessive worry about finances and health, difficulty with sleeping and concentrating, weight changes, a loss of interest in personal hygiene and appearance, and withdrawal from regular social activities

As with other illnesses, depression has various types and levels. A recent study published in *Cognitive Therapy and Research* reported that late-onset depression (in people over 60) can affect the brain's *executive functions*—planning and control—and can spiral into excessive *rumination*—uncontrolled thought patterns that are repetitive, negative, and destructive. Symptoms include inattention, a decline in memory, rigid thinking, and a lack of inhibition.

Depression is sometimes difficult to diagnose in older people. To avoid being considered weak or crazy, older people often complain of physical pain to their doctor, rather than admitting to feelings of hopelessness and worthlessness, loss of interest, or prolonged grief.

Depression can become so severe that the senior feels compelled to anesthetize himself with drugs or alcohol. Alcoholism among older people is considered a "hidden epidemic." The very symptoms that would suggest a problem are ignored or misdiagnosed because they are also associated with aging—such symptoms might include dizziness and falls, incontinence and poor hygiene, confusion and impaired memory, depression, and excessive napping, disinterest in food, and isolation.

The typical consequences of alcohol abuse—including family and financial problems, job loss, and arrest—are not really a deterrent for an older person. People who are retired, drive less, and live at a distance from family and friends, are able to drink alone for a long time before the problem is detected. It finally becomes obvious to the family when the aging alcoholic can no longer function independently.

The Center for Substance Abuse Treatment reported that 15 percent of male alcoholics and 24 percent of females began abusing alcohol between the ages of 60–69, and 14 percent of men and 28 percent of women began abusing it between the ages of 70–79. Social isolation, loss and grief, housing and financial concerns, and physical and mental health problems are some of the reasons for late-life drinking.

Because of the physiologic changes associated with aging and the pharmacologic effect of mixing medications with alcohol, people 65 and older are especially vulnerable to the adverse effects of abuse. Their immune systems are compromised, and their ability to resist disease is greatly diminished.

Education is key before intervention can be successful. See *Aging and Addiction: Helping Older Adults Overcome Alcohol or Medication Dependence* by Carol Colleran and Debra Jay for more information (published by Hazelden). Visit the National Institutes of Health at www.niaaa.nih.gov. Call Focus on Recovery at 800-234-0420 for program referrals, or call Alcoholics Anonymous at 800-593-3330.

Confront the problem with love, compassion, and understanding. Visit a physician for a proper diagnosis, and take heart. Generally, older people stay in recovery programs and respond well to treatment.

Holidays can also be difficult for seniors. They are generally a special time for family members to gather, express their love, and pass on cherished traditions to new generations. Most of us anticipate and treasure these moments and the people with whom we share them. It's perfectly understandable to feel mournful and even heartbroken when we suffer their loss or the loss of others with whom to celebrate.

Normally, feelings of sadness during the holidays are temporary and don't impact our ability to function. However, it is important to consult a physician about the possibility of depression if the sadness is so great that the senior withdraws from regular activities, or experiences a lack of energy, inability to concentrate, or a change in eating or sleeping patterns.

Clinical depression, which can also be caused by biochemical changes in the brain, interferes with performing the simplest tasks, erodes self-esteem, and can cause the affected person to question the value of life.

The good news is that treatment, including behavioral changes and medication, is highly effective, even dramatically so among seniors. Treatment should be carefully monitored and results vary, but usually marked improvement occurs in 4–12 weeks.

Talk therapy is also beneficial. Seniors should surround themselves with supportive people who understand and sympathize, and they should seek out a good therapist. Contact the American Association for Geriatric Psychiatry (AAGP) at 301-654-7850 or visit www.aagponline.org to request board-certified experts in your area. When properly diagnosed and treated, more than 80 percent of people who suffer from depression recover fully and return to normal, productive lives.

# FEAR

Fear is a common reaction to aging. Seniors are afraid of being institutionalized, being left in the care of strangers, and being left alone and vulnerable. They have good cause to worry.

It's difficult and painful to imagine anyone harming those who are frail, ill, and totally dependent on others. The trust given by families to assisted living centers, rehabilitation facilities, and nursing homes is sacred but often broken, and don't let the décor fool you. Some of the worst cases of fraud, neglect, and abuse have occurred in the plushest surroundings.

The National Elder Abuse Study reported that over 500,000 Americans, 60 years and older, were abused in 1996. The study also revealed that only 16 percent of these cases were reported and referred for help. The Senate Special Committee of Aging now estimates there are 5 million victims every year.

According to Dr. Linda Woolf of Webster University, there are six types of abuse, each of which causes specific symptoms:

- ▶ *Neglect.* Malnourishment, chronic physical and psychiatric problems, dehydration, bed sores, and poor hygiene.
- ▶ *Physical trauma.* Scratches, bruises, cut, burns, punctures, choke marks; evidence of restraint, such as rope burns, gag marks, and welts; repeated and unexplained injury, including sprains, fractures, detached retina, and paralysis; inconsistent explanations of injuries; and a lag time between incident and treatment.
- ▶ *Psychological.* Passivity, shame, anxiety, depression, confusion, trembling, cowering, clinging, or lack of eye contact.

▶ *Sexual abuse.* Trauma to the genital area, venereal disease, infections, discharge, odor, and psychological symptoms, including the above.

▶ *Financial.* Bank statements diverted, accounts changed from one bank to another, documents drawn up for an elder no longer competent to sign, and missing property.

▶ *Basic rights.* Withholding mail, obstructing religious freedom, over-medicating or sedating, and preventing the elder from speaking.

If you recognize any of these symptoms, call 911 and report your suspicions immediately. You can also contact your local Adult Protective Service (APS), and someone from the agency will assign a caseworker to investigate (usually within 24 hours) and intervene as necessary. Contact Eldercare Locator at 800-677-1116 for the number in your area, and visit www.elderabusecenter.org for a list of hotlines, which are free, anonymous, and confidential.

## GRIEF

Loss and the grief it causes is another major component of growing older. First, children leave home to begin their own lives. Although parents understand the need and naturalness of this process, the emotional response is often grief.

Later, seniors begin to lose family members and friends to illness and death, and their grief becomes even more profound because their own and their spouse's mortality comes into question as well.

The final loss is that of a spouse or even a child. Family members can be well-meaning, but unaware of how difficult and painful it is to cope with such deaths. Such a profound loss causes extreme mental anguish and a flood of feelings—shock, sorrow, anger, guilt, depression, fear, and even desperation, depending on the extent to which daily life is changed.

Professionals are just beginning to understand the effect of grief on the mind and body, but studies show that it's crucial to acknowledge feelings if recovery is to take place. Allow yourself to mourn for your loved one and yourself. Don't be afraid to cry, scream, and be angry. The more you experience your feelings, the easier it will be to let them go.

Discuss your feelings, particularly with others who feel the same way. Contact the funeral home, Hospice (800-658-8898), and the American Association of Retired People (AARP; 888-687-2277 or visit www.aarp.org/life/griefandloss) for information about recovery programs and support groups for people who are grieving. You'll feel understood and encouraged, and you will learn skills to help you cope with your loss. See *The Grief Recovery Handbook: A Step-by-Step Program for Moving Beyond Loss* by John W. James for more information.

*Statistics indicate that widows and widowers are at higher risk for illness, so take care of your physical health. Discuss changes in your well-being with your doctor. Avoid numbing the pain with drugs or alcohol, and get some exercise.*

Statistics indicate that widows and widowers are at higher risk for illness, so take care of your physical health. Discuss changes in your well-being with your doctor. Avoid numbing the pain with drugs or alcohol, and get some exercise. Although cooking for one and eating alone can be painful reminders, it's crucial to not skip meals. Share shopping and cooking chores with a single friend or neighbor.

As your grief becomes less powerful, your strength for moving forward will grow. See *Seven Choices: Taking the Steps to a New Life After Losing Someone You Love* by Elizabeth H. Neeld for help in healing and forging your new identity.

## CARING CONVERSATIONS AT THE END OF LIFE

Of all the phases of life that we experience, the end of life is the one for which we are least prepared, yet preparation is crucial to ensuring that our wishes are respected and in determining how our final days will be spent.

Take the time you need to evaluate your life, mend fences, handle regrets, and finish any unfinished business. Also, making final decisions lessens the physical, psychological, and social suffering for everyone involved.

The Center for Practical Bioethics has an excellent workbook called *Caring Conversations* that can be downloaded from www.practicalbioethics.org, or ordered by calling 800-344-3829. Using a series of questions, it guides you through the process of identifying your beliefs and preferences in the areas of spiritual/religious values, health care, career and work, financial matters, and personal relationships.

Some examples of the decisions that you might be guided to make, and ultimately share with your family, are:

▶ Deciding what will make you feel most comforted during illness
▶ Whether you want to live your last days in a hospital, a hospice, or at home
▶ End-of-life treatments, such as pain medication but not tube feeding
▶ Wills and powers of attorney
▶ Fulfilling financial obligations, such as a prepaid funeral and trusts to pay medical bills

Read *Dying Well* by Dr. Ira Byock, who suggests that dying people need to say, "I forgive you. Please forgive me. I love you. Thank you and good-bye."

Perhaps the kindest and most respectful farewell is allowing the opportunity for these caring conversations.

## IMPORTANT END-OF-LIFE DOCUMENTS

If you hope to control your quality of life during your last days, preparing for them is not only responsible but critical. According to Attorney

Rick B. Weaver, an elder law specialist who can be reached by e-mail at rweaver@shannongracey.com, "each person should consider signing three documents":

- ▶ A Directive to Physicians (giving the family directions when the person is on life support with no chance of recovery)
- ▶ A Medical Power of Attorney (appointing an agent to make medical decisions if the person is incapacitated)
- ▶ A Do Not Resuscitate Order (done when a person is in extremely poor health and does not want to be resuscitated in a medical emergency)

The agent and back-up agent on the Medical Power of Attorney are important designations. They are similar to the executor of a will. If a person appoints someone as a medical agent who is not committed to carrying out the person's wishes, problems can result in the same way as when an executor fails to carry out the terms of a will.

The decision about whether or not to receive artificial feeding and hydration is becoming a bigger issue each year. If a person does not want artificial feeding and hydration, this should be set forth in the Physician's Directive.

If a person does not want to be revived, it's critical that he sign a Do Not Resuscitate Order and keep it in close proximity. Otherwise, it's possible that emergency medical personnel might revive the patient against his wishes.

## HOSPICE

Refusing food, losing weight, sleeping more, and talking less are sometimes indicators of the beginning of the end, but no one has a crystal ball, and doctors will be the first to say so. All the family can do is ensure that their loved one's health and comfort is optimum.

Hospice is an excellent program that is underutilized and often begun so late in the process that many beneficial services go unused. Although the purpose of hospice is to provide compassionate support and extraordinary care for people in the final phase of a terminal illness, the program's goal is to enhance the quality of life regardless of its duration.

The hospice team often includes a medical director, physician, nurse, certified nurse assistant (CNA), social worker, spiritual care coordinator, therapist, and counselor. The team members subscribe to a holistic approach. Volunteers provide companionship and emotional support to the patient and respite services for the caregivers, including shopping, errands, childcare, and preparing light meals.

Begin by discussing the senior's condition with her doctor, who must certify to hospice staff that she is no longer thriving or that her disease is terminal. Ask the physician to recommend the best hospice provider; call the National Hospice Organization at 800-658-8898; or visit www.nhpco.org for valuable information and recommendations.

Once a patient has been examined, records reviewed, and medications evaluated, a care plan will be developed. Then hospice will provide all necessary equipment, supplies, and medicines—whether the patient is at home or in a facility—and Medicare, Medicaid, or private insurance will cover the cost.

The final phase of the journey need not be feared. With help and support, the last moments in our loved one's life can be serene and uplifting. It can be a time for family members to gather, to share memories, and to give comfort to each other. It can be a time to celebrate someone's life and legacy. Saying goodbye to a loved one in this way brings closure and peace.

# Gratitude

## *Honoring Those We Love*

*Dear Ageless:*

*My father was married for 52 years, had a wonderful career, and fathered his three children well. Five strokes stole his ability to walk, swallow, and read—his favorite pastime. I'd like to help him stay positive, but his present condition seems to eclipse all that was good in his life. How can we refocus and find something for which to be grateful?*

*Hoping to help Dad*

*Dear Hoping:*

*Although you can't fully grasp the magnitude of your father's feelings, treat him with as much empathy as possible. People are far more receptive to change when their present circumstances are understood and validated.*

*Your father's losses have been great, so expect some of the same grief stages people experience when a loved one dies— denial, anger, and depression—emotions that can hinder making even the most beneficial changes. Be sure he's had a complete examination and that appropriate medication has been prescribed.*

*Prevent isolation and inactivity. Discourage too much sleep, daydreaming, and watching television. They are as much an escape as alcohol or drugs. Taking action is the best remedy.*

*Begin projects that don't require the skills he's lost—a new hobby, a coin or stamp collection, puzzles and crafts. Attend worship services regularly and take field trips to museums, the theater, or the library. Check out books on tape for listening and discussing with your dad.*

*Set an example of gratitude for him, and express how much you appreciate all he's done for you. Be very specific about how his help and guidance has impacted your life. Ask him to share his stories—the mentors in his life, the pivotal moments, and his best and most memorable times. Suggest writing them down in a gratitude journal and reading them aloud periodically. Read "Simple Abundance" by Sarah Ban Breathnach for inspiration.*

*Encourage him to honor his past by writing letters of gratitude to family and friends. Expressing appreciation and focusing on the blessings can impact attitude, create a sense of well-being, and produce peace of mind.*

*Ageless*

Children take comfort in the thought that their parents—the only real heroes in most people's lives—will always be sturdy, vibrant, and completely competent. Parents symbolize security, the rock from which children draw strength and endurance.

It's heartbreaking to see these idols decline into illness, pain, insecurity, and dependence. Even adult children struggle when the rock begins to break into pieces. This is when they must accept, perhaps for the first time, their parents' mortality—and their own.

This is also when roles are reversed, and parents become those who need caregiving. Aged parents are forced to relinquish their power and independence and look to their children for survival. It can be terrifying.

Children must begin to take responsibility for the care of their dependent parents and the hard work this entails, but they must do so in a way that protects their parent's dignity. Understanding is the first step. Honor your parents' feelings with an attentive ear and great empathy. They will feel more secure if they know their concerns are important to you, and that they have an advocate in their corner.

Protect a senior's rights by involving them in the decisions that will affect their lives. Be sure their desires are expressed in legal documents, including a Last Will and Testament, funeral and burial preferences, a Living Will or Physician's Directive, a Power of Attorney, and a Durable Power of Attorney. Visit www.caregiver.com for information and resources. Aging parents can find solace in knowing they are prepared and protected.

*Protect a senior's rights by involving them in the decisions that will affect their lives. Be sure their desires are expressed in legal documents, including a Last Will and Testament, funeral and burial preferences, a Living Will or Physician's Directive, a Power of Attorney, and a Durable Power of Attorney. Visit www.caregiver.com for information and resources. Aging parents can find solace in knowing they are prepared and protected.*

## Show Your Gratitude

Caring for older parents is a blessing, a repayment for their sacrifices, and an opportunity to express the deepest feelings in words and action. It's a true labor of love and an opportunity to say "Thank you."

Gratitude doesn't have to come in the form of material "things." In fact, people who are past middle age rarely need much. Ironically, we spend the first half of life accumulating things and the second half figuring out how to give them away. Generally, the best gift is what our parents gave us—time and attention.

If people really considered it, the job description for the role of mother (on-call 24 hours a day, 7 days a week for no salary or health benefits) would send most intelligent people running. No one would want the job. For their constant care and self-sacrifice, Moms ask little in return—only respect, appreciation, and remembrance. This can't happen, though, if they're left alone. Assess your mom's (or dad's) ability to live independently. Perhaps it's time to ask her how she would feel about living with her children or having extended visits with them.

If she's interested, the best plan is to have her live with one sibling and have long visits with the others. She will think of her primary residence as her home, with all the physical and emotional security that ensures.

If such a plan is not possible, devise a reasonable schedule for moving her from the home of one child to another. This way, the responsibility for her care and attention can be divided—and the benefits of multigenerational living are many, especially for grandchildren.

Moving from place to place can be difficult, even for young people, so be considerate about the time frame for her visits. Each stay should be significant enough in length that she will not think she's being shuttled around.

## GIFTS FOR MOMS

Your words of love and regular visits are the most meaningful and best-remembered gifts. If your Mom is fine living independently, consider planning a family reunion with all of her children and their families. Give her a video of the event. An embroidered or calligraphic family tree and a family portrait for her wall would be valued gifts, so be sure to have a photographer present. Visit www.allmothersdaygifts.com, www.everythingmothersday.com, and www.theholidayspot.com/mothersday (or call 800-326-6626) for a variety of lovely keepsakes and personalized gifts.

You might also give her certificates for a day of pampering—a manicure, pedicure, and hair styling at her favorite salon, and facials, wraps, and massages at a spa. Then whisk her off to the theater for a live production, dress-up dining, and a hotel stay, or to a charming cottage or quaint bed-and-breakfast for a weekend of sightseeing or scrap-booking.

If she's not able to travel long distances, take her to brunch before church, lunch at a tearoom, and antiquing or shopping. Remember to buy her a corsage to wear for the holidays.

## Gifts for Dads

Senior Dads deserve some thought, creativity, and care, too. After all, they put their own needs on hold, sometimes indefinitely, worked a lifetime to provide for their families, and sacrificed their own dreams to ensure those of their children.

Send him a loving e-mail or call before Father's Day or his birthday, and tell him you'd like to arrange a day for just the two of you—a picnic at the botanic gardens, a game at the ballpark, a car trip to a place he's never been, or a day doing something he loves.

Fix his favorite meal, mow his lawn, clean out the garage, and offer to take care of his house and pets, so he and your Mom can have a special weekend or take a trip.

If your Dad is housebound, plant a fruit or flowering bush and hang a bird feeder outside his window. He'll enjoy the coming and going of the birds and keep interested in the growth process.

As people grow older, photos take on greater meaning, particularly for those who struggle with short-term memory loss. Five minutes ago may be a fog, but the distant past is remembered with crystal clarity. Make thematic scrapbooks of various special events through the years or frame a collage of his favorite pictures.

Instead of a card, write a letter that expresses appreciation in a very specific manner. Highlight special moments you shared, and recall the times that made all the difference in your life. He will cherish it forever.

## GIFT CARDS

Gift cards have become a popular solution because the stigma of these cards being a lazy person's way of giving is gone. Gift cards are readily available at restaurants, malls, grocery stores, and a variety of retailers. They are simple to buy, reduce shopping time, and alleviate guesswork. They also allow the recipient to buy whatever she wants or needs within a time frame that allows her to take advantage of sales.

There are drawbacks. The cards are easy to lose, sometimes stolen, and they are often allowed to expire. Fees and restrictions erode their value, and buyers aren't protected by regulations. In a letter to the Federal Trade Commission, Representative Joe Barton wrote, "Consumers will be confused by the different rules that retailers have for their cards, and some have been and will be deceived about card restrictions."

To avoid difficulty, buy from a reputable merchant, and avoid the fraudulent cards often sold on the Internet. Consider a gift card from the local pharmacy, gas station, bookstore, or favorite restaurant. The likelihood that the card will be used is greater.

Some gift cards carry inactivity fees that reduce the card's value, or maintenance fees that can be as high as a one-time assessment of $25 or $4.95 a month. Other cards expire in 6 months, and some merchants tack on a surcharge, which means a $25 gift card could cost you as much as $35. Be informed and purchase such a card carefully.

Explain all the gift card restrictions to the recipient, and include a copy of the receipt (especially if the recipient's memory is not what it once was) when giving the card. It will be easier to get a replacement if the gift card is lost or stolen.

## Gifts That Last a Lifetime

Life is finite. The only real fact is that we will die (some people really do get out of paying taxes); and although we believe we will always remember our loved ones, the truth is that our memories fade, even of our parents and grandparents.

Photos are a lovely, quick reminder, but nothing equals seeing the expressions and hearing the voices of those we love. Take the time to interview the people who are close to you before it's too late. Develop a list of questions, pull out the video camera, and ask the most important people in your life to tell you their story—to share their joys and sorrows, the history of their own lives and that of the family, and their favorite memories.

StoryCorps, an organization that preserves this kind of historical data, can help. Founded by Dave Isay of Sound Portraits Production (the parent company) in October, 2003, StoryCorps has conducted and archived over 5,000 oral histories. Modeled after a 1930s program in a section of President Franklin Roosevelt's New Deal, which hired unemployed writers to document oral history and folklore throughout the United States, StoryCorps is "a national project intended to instruct and inspire people to record each others' stories in sound."

StoryCorps is in the process of building soundproof recording studios across the country, and, as of this writing, they offer two permanent locations in New York City called *StoryBooths* and two traveling studios called *MobileBooths*. A trained facilitator aids in question development suited to the person being interviewed, handles all the technical aspects of the recording, produces the CD (a digital recording with broadcast-quality equipment), and archives the 40-minute interview with the American Folklife Center at the Library of Congress.

This is an extraordinary value, because only a $10 donation is requested. The actual $200 cost is underwritten by various organizations, including the Corporation for Public Broadcasting and National

Public Radio, which broadcasts the interviews. StoryCorps is also supported by public generosity.

The process is simple: Choose an interview partner, who must be over 10 years old, make a reservation online at www.storycorps.net, or call 800-850-4406 (24 hours/7 days a week), develop a list of questions, and arrive 10 minutes before your scheduled time to conduct the interview or tell your own story.

If you live too far from a StoryBooth or MobileBooth, visit http://storycorps.net to download a *Do It Yourself Guide* that lists equipment needed and outlines the complete process for conducting a StoryCorps interview, including questions, tips, and an interview checklist. Read *Flophouse*, a book based on the Sound Portraits Production radio stories by Dave Isay, for inspiration.

> *A memory is a valuable piece of history. Sharing your memories with the generations of people who will follow you is a precious gift.*

A memory is a valuable piece of history. Sharing your memories with the generations of people who will follow you is a precious gift.

Gratitude is one of the greatest gifts of all. Be sure to *show it* to your spouse. With care and perseverance, a happy marriage is possible. When you give your spouse what he or she needs emotionally, generally, the favor will be returned many-fold.

## GIFTS FOR WIVES

Showing your wife how much you love her will help create and sustain a successful marriage. Most women long to feel cherished, and it's rarely about the gift or how much is spent. Thought and effort make a woman feel valued.

Write her a love letter. Chronicle the special times in your marriage, describe the qualities that make her extraordinary, and thank her for all she's done to make your life special. Personalize the salutation with an endearment and close with a promise of enduring love.

Use special stationery, spray it with cologne, and put it on her pillow so she finds it in the morning. Your words will be a blessing then, and a comfort to her in the future whenever she rereads your letter.

Tell her you've planned a special day for just the two of you—perhaps the plan might include an outing to a fair, art show, or museum, a concert in the park, or a drive in the country. Pack a picnic lunch, a thermos of homemade cappuccino or hot chocolate, blankets, and lawn chairs. Be sure to stop and watch the sunset.

Cook dinner for her. Even if you're not the best chef in the kitchen, simple fare served beautifully will be remembered. Don't forget candles (lots of little ones floating in a glass bowl are romantic), fresh flowers, and music you can dance to afterward. Have her favorite movie ready to watch together that evening and hold hands. You will have orchestrated a day she will never forget, and said "I love you" with your every action.

## GIFTS FOR HUSBANDS

Consider giving your husband a day of his favorite activities, which might include meals, music, and merriment. Wake him with a festive breakfast tray. Add a photo album of all your special moments together and a scented love letter from the heart. Chronicle the pivotal times in your marriage; describe the qualities that make him your hero and thank him for all he's done to make your life special. Your letter will be a blessing then, and heartwarming in the future whenever he rereads it.

If writing isn't your forté, consider giving a personalized poem or telegram sung live over the telephone. Visit www.poetspassion.com for various selections and www.songsender.com for an original song that can be funny or sentimental. Choose from a variety of musical styles including Big Band and Romantic Ballads.

Try shopping on the Internet for economical and unique gifts, such as a basket of chocolates, gourmet cookies, or other delectable snacks. Visit www.wiredseniors.com and www.giftideasforseniors.com for gadgets, aides, and games.

Have little gifts delivered throughout the day for one surprise after another. End by giving him a Memory-a-Day Book (purchased from www.seniorstore.com), in which he'll answer questions like "What's your favorite memory?" and "Do you have a piece of good advice?" Tell him it will become a family heirloom cherished by the family he's created. You'll have given him a day of feeling important, honored, and loved.

It takes only a small amount of effort to show our love and appreciation for the people who are most important in our lives. Yet, our gifts will be remembered for a lifetime, and beyond to future generations. Take the time to show others you care. Sometimes, even the smallest gift is the most treasured.

# Resources

## Chapter 1
## Aging Gracefully: *The Power of the Mind—Body—Spirit Connection*

### Books

Adler, Jack. *Splendid Seniors*. Nashville: Pearlsong Press, 2007.

Crowley, Chris and Henry S. Lodge. *Younger Next Year: A Guide to Living Like 50 Until You're 80 and Beyond*. New York: Workman Publishing Co., 2004.

Cutler, Howard C., and the Dalai Lama. *The Art of Happiness: A Handbook for Living*. New York: Simon & Schuster Publishing, 2000.

Fries, James F. *Aging Well: A Guide for Successful Seniors*. Boston: Perseus Books, 1989.

Firestone, Lisa, Firestone, Robert W., and Catlett, Joyce. *Conquer Your Critical Inner Voice: A Revolutionary Program to Counter Negative Thoughts*. San Francisco: New Harbinger Publications, Inc., 2002.

McKhann, Guy and Marilyn Albert. *Keep Your Brain Young: The Complete Guide to Physical and Emotional Health and Longevity*. New York: Wiley Publishing, 2002.

Petty, David L. *Aging Gracefully: Keeping Joy in the Journey*. Nashville: Broadman and Holman Publishers, 2003.

Sandford, John and Paula. *The Transformation of the Inner Man, The Most Comprehensive Book on Inner Healing Today*. New York: Charisma House, 2006.

Segal, Irene. *Exploring Coaching*. Boulder, CO: LearnMore Publishing, 2004.

Wei, Jeanne Y., and Sue Levkoff. *Aging Well: The Complete Guide to Physical and Emotional Health*. New York: John Wiley & Sons, 2000.

Weil, Andrew. *Healthy Aging: A Lifelong Guide to Your Physical and Spiritual Well-Being*, New York: Knopf Publishing, 2005.

Yount, David. *Celebrating the Rest of Your Life: A Baby Boomer's Guide to Spirituality*, Minneapolis: Augsburg Books, 2005.

### Websites

American Association of Retired People: www.aarp.org/health
www.allaboutprayer.com
www.educate-yourself.org
www.emofree.com
www.explorefaith.org

www.familydoctor.org/famdocen/home/seniors
www.library.thinkquest.org
www.nihseniorhealth.gov
www.seniorhealth.com
www.webmd.com

## Chapter 2
### Food as Potent Medicine: *Nutrition for a Zestful Life*
**Books**

Arthritis Foundation (Tennessee Chapter). *Help Yourself—Recipes and Resources from The Arthritis Foundation.* Author, 2000.

Barnard, Neal. *Foods That Fight Pain: Revolutionary New Strategies for Maximum Pain Relief.* New York: Three Rivers Press, 1999.

Black, Jessica K. *The Anti-Inflammation Diet and Recipe Book.* Alameda, CA: Hunter House, 2006.

Felix, Clara. *FAQ's All About Omega-3 Oils.* New York: Avery Publishing Group Inc., 2002.

Hensrud, Donald. *Mayo Clinic on Healthy Weight for Everybody.* Rochester, MN: Mayo Clinic, 2005.

Holford, Patrick. *The New Optimum Nutrition Bible.* Berkeley, CA: Crossing Press, 2004.

Lindsay, Anne. *Anne Lindsay's Light Kitchen.* New York: John Wiley & Sons, 2002.

Napier, Kristine. *Power Nutrition for Your Chronic Illness.* New York: Macmillan, 1998.

Oxmoor House. *Cooking Light Five Star Recipes: The Best of 10 Years.* Atlanta, GA: Leisure Arts, 1997.

Oz, Mehmet C., and Michael F. Roizen. *You on a Diet: The Insider's Guide to Easy and Permanent Weight Loss.* New York: HarperCollins, 2007.

Prevention Magazine Editors. *The 'Prevention' Lose Weight Guidebook.* New York: Rodale Press, 2006.

Prevention Magazine Editors. *The Sugar Solution Cookbook: More Than 200 Delicious Recipes to Balance Your Blood Sugar Naturally.* New York: Rodale Press, 2006.

Richard, Sandi. *Life's on Fire: Cooking for the Rushed.* New York: Scribner, 2007.

Rinzler, Carol Ann. *Nutrition for Dummies.* Indianapolis: Wiley Publishing, 2006.

Saltzman, Edward, and R.D. McQuillian. *The Complete Idiot's Guide to Losing Weight.* Santa Monica, CA: Alpha Communications, 1997.

Sass, Loma J. *The New Soy Cookbook: Tempting Recipes for Soybeans, Soy Milk, Tofu, Tempeh, Miso and Soy Sauce.* San Francisco: Chronicle Books, 1998.

Sears, Barry. *The Soy Zone: 101 Delicious and Easy-to-Prepare Recipes.* New York: HarperCollins, 2001.

Simopoulos, Artemis P., and Jo Robinson. *The Omega Plan: The Medically Proven Diet That Gives You the Essential Nutrients You Need.* New York: HarperCollins, 1998.

University of Alabama Research Foundation. *Essential Arthritis Cookbook.* Mankato, MN: Appletree Press, 1999.

Weight Watchers. *Cook It Quick!* New York: Fireside Publishing, 2002.

Weil, Andrew. *Eating Well for Optimum Health: The Essential Guide to Bringing Health and Pleasure Back to Eating.* New York: HarperCollins, 2001.

Wernick, Sarah, and Miriam Nelson. *Strong Women Stay Slim.* New York: Bantam Books, 1998.

Willett, Walter C. *Eat, Drink, and Be Healthy: The Harvard Medical School Guide to Healthy Eating.* New York: Free Press, 2005.

## Websites

American Dietetic Association: www.eatright.org

American Heart Association: www.americanheart.org

Dietary Guidelines for Americans: www.healthierus.gov/dietaryguidelines

Food and Drug Administration: www.fda.gov

Institute of Food Technologists: www.ift.org

Institute of Medicine Food and Nutrition Board: www.iom.edu

National Institutes of Health, Office of Dietary Supplements: www.ods.od.nih.gov

United States Department of Agriculture: www.usda.gov

United States Department of Agriculture: www.mypyramid.gov

## Chapter 3
## Spice Up Your Diet: *Antioxidants for an Anti-Aging Lifestyle*

### Books

Bealer, Bonnie, and Alan Bennett Weinberg. *The World of Caffeine.* New York: Routledge, 2002.

Bhide, Monica. *The Spice Is Right: Easy Indian Cooking for Today.* New York: Callawind Publications, 2002.

Busch, Felecia. *The New Nutrition: From Antioxidants to Zucchini.* New York: Wiley Publishing, 2000.

Farrington, Karen. *Herbs and Spices: A Gourmet's Guide.* London: Carlton Books, 1999.

McDowall, Anne. *Herbs and Spices.* London: Salamander Books Limited, 1996.

Murdock, Linda. *A Busy Cook's Guide to Spices: How to Introduce New Flavors to Everyday Meals.* London: Bellwether Books, 2001.

Page, Linda. *Cooking for Healthy Healing: Food Is Your Pharmacy.* Del Ray Oaks, CA: Healthy Healing Inc., 2002.

Peter, K.V. *Handbook of Herbs and Spices.* Boca Raton, FL: CRC Press LLC, 2004.

Simonds, Nina. *Spices of Life: Simple and Delicious Recipes for Great Health.* New York: Alfred A. Knopf Publishers, 2005.

Simonds, Nina. *A Spoonful of Ginger: Irresistible, Health-Giving Recipes from Asian Kitchens.* New York: Alfred A. Knopf Publishers, 1999.

Tull, Anita. *Food and Nutrition.* Oxford, UK: Oxford University Press, 1996.

Woodruff, Sandra. *The Best-Kept Secrets of Healthy Cooking.* New York: Avery Publishing, 2000.

## Websites

www.101cookbooks.com

www.activegourmetholidays.com

www.chef2chef.net

www.chilepepperinstitute.org

www.epicurious.com

www.healinggourmet.com

www.nikibone.com/recipe/salad_dressings.html

www.saveur.com

www.spicycooking.com

www.visualrecipes.com

## Chapter 4
## Move That Body: *The Best Prescription for Healthy Aging*
## Books

Bacso, Stanley, and Christopher Oswald. *Stretching For Fitness, Health & Performance: The Complete Handbook for All Ages & Fitness Levels.* New York: Sterling Publishing, 2003.

Burns, George. *How to Live to be 100 or More: The Ultimate Diet, Sex, and Exercise Book.* Boston: G.K. Hall & Co., 1986.

Coulter, David H. *Anatomy of Hatha Yoga: A Manual for Students, Teachers and Practitioners,* Indianapolis: Body and Breath Inc., 2001.

Devi, Joy Nischala. *The Healing Path of Yoga: Time-Honored Wisdom and Scientifically Proven Methods That Alleviate Stress, Open Your Heart, and Enrich Your Life.* New York: Three Rivers Press, 2000.

Fekete, Michael. *Strength Training for Seniors: How to Rewind Your Biological Clock.* Alameda, CA: Hunter House, 2006.

Fried, Robert. *Breathe Well; Be Well.* New York: Wiley Publishing, 1999.

Goto, Kazushige, et al. Enhancement of fat metabolism by repeated bouts of moderate endurance exercise. *Journal of Applied Physiology,* June 2007; 102: 2158–2164.

Grout, Pam. *Jumpstart Your Metabolism: How to Lose Weight by Changing the Way You Breathe.* New York: Fireside Publishers, 1998.

Hale, Teresa. *Breathing Free: The Revolutionary 5-Day Program to Heal Asthma, Emphysema, Bronchitis and Other Respiratory Ailments.* New York: Three Rivers Press, 2000.

Hamilton, Mina. *Serenity to Go: Calming Techniques for Your Hectic Life.* New York: New Harbinger Publications, 2001.

Hendricks, Gay. *Conscious Breathing: Breathwork for Health, Stress Release, and Person Mastery.* New York: Bantam Books, 1995.

Jahnke, Roger. *The Healing Promise of Qi: Creating Extraordinary Wellness through Qigong and Tai Chi.* New York: McGraw-Hill, 2002.

Lewis, Dennis. *Breathing as a Metaphor for Living: Teachings and Exercises on Complete and Natural Breathing.* A two-cassette audio-tape program. Louisville, CO: Sounds True, 1998.

Lewis, Dennis. *Free Your Breath, Free Your Life.* Boston: Shambhala Press, 2004.

Miller, Fred. *How to Calm Down: Three Deep Breaths to Peace of Mind.* New York: Grand Central Publishing, 2003.

Morgan, David, and Jon Griswold. *Basic Training: A Fundamental Guide to Fitness for Men.* New York: St. Martin's Griffin, 2000.

National Institute on Aging. Call 800-222-2225 to order their exercise video and guidebook.

Talbott, Shawn. *The Cortisol Connection.* Alameda, CA: Hunter House, 2007.

Scott, John C. *Ashtanga Yoga: The Definitive Step-by-Step Guide to Dynamic Yoga.* New York: Three Rivers Press, 2001.

Shaw, Scott. *The Little Book of Yoga Breathing: Pranayama Made Easy.* Newburyport, ME: Red Wheel/Weiser, 2004.

Weil, Andrew. *Breathing: The Master Key to Self Healing*, an audio product read by Andrew Weil. Louisville, CO: Sounds True, 2000.

Wilson, Stanley D. *Qi Gong for Beginners: Eight Easy Movements for Vibrant Health*, Photographs by Barry Kaplan. New York: Sterling Publications, 1999.

Zi, Nancy. *The Art of Breathing: Six Simple Lessons to Improve Performance, Health, and Well-Being.* Berkeley, CA: Frog Ltd., 2000.

## Websites

www.airportgyms.com

www.bestbreathingexercises.com—Karen Van Ness

www.cathe.com

www.cooperaerobics.com

www.crossfit.com

www.fitday.com

www.fitwatch.com

www.infofaq.com/buying-online/personal/exercise-videos/reviews.html

www.jumpUSA.com
www.letsexercise.com
www.lifetimefitness.com
www.mydietexercise.com
www.nihseniorhealth.gov
www.onlinepersonaltrainer.co.uk/essentialwebsites.htm
www.productivefitness.com
www.runnersworld.com
www.swiminfo.com
www.triathletemag.com
www.velonews.com

## Chapter 5
## Hitting the Road: *See the World Without Breaking the Bank*

### Books

Doyle, Patrick J. *New Travelers Health Guide.* Camarillo, CA: Devorss & Co., 2001.

Gilbert, Verne E. *Senior Sporting Adventures.* Smokey Mountain Press, 2003.

Harrington, Candy B. *101 Accessible Vacations.* New York: Demos Medical Publishing, 2008.

Harrington, Candy B. *There Is Room at the Inn.* New York: Demos Medical Publishing, 2006.

Harrington, Candy B. *Barrier Free Travel.* New York: Demos Medical Publishing, 2005.

Health Ideas. *Anyone Can Travel: The Essential Guide for Seniors, People with Disabilities.* Health Problems and All Travelers. Victoria, BC, Canada: Trafford Publishing, 2000.

Moeller, Bill, and Jan Moeller. *Complete Guide to Full-time RVing: Life on the Open Road.* Ventura, CA: TL Enterprises, Inc., 1998.

Ronald, Robert B. *Seniors & Disabled Passengers.* Indianapolis: IADC Publishing, 2001.

Toland, James. *Travel Tips & Trips for Seniors.* Little Rock, AK: Bridgeway Press, 2002.

Weintz, Walter. *Discount Guide for Travelers Over 55.* New York: EP Dutton, 2001.

White, Phil and Carol White. *Live Your Road Trip Dream: Travel for a Year for the Cost of Staying Home.* Wilsonville, OR: RLI Press, 2004.

### Websites

www.50plusexpeditions.com
Adventure travel for people over 50 who want to explore the globe.

www.adventuresabroad.com/category/goldenyears.jsp

*Adventures Abroad* features international work, study opportunities, and travel-related issues for people of various ages.

www.amtrak.com

Call Amtrak at (800) USA-RAIL to arrange train travel.

www.bedandbreakfast.com

View and virtually visit various B&Bs. Over 6,500 are noted.

www.caretaker.org

See *The Caretaker Gazette.* Published since 1983, it's the only publication in the world dedicated to the property caretaking field.

www.frommers.com

Arthur Frommer features a specific section on senior travel and includes information about traveling on a budget.

www.cstn.org

*Connecting, Solo Travel News* offers a bimonthly newsletter, a comprehensive website, and a Travel Directory. Six issues of the newsletter, a copy of the annual single-friendly directory, unlimited travel companion advertising in the newsletter, and access to online advice is available to new members. Offers a free catalog. The business is located at 11 Avenue de Lafayette, Boston, MA 02111-1746; phone: 877-426-8056.

www.dotcr.ost.dot.gov/asp/airacc.asp

Air Carrier Access Act that addresses the rights of the disabled

www.elderhostel.org

Elderhostel; phone: 877-426-8056

www.eldertrav.com

ElderTrav.com is a website about adventure travel for seniors.

www.eldertreks.com

Eldertreks is the first travel company designed exclusively for people 50 and over. They offer small-group adventures in over 50 countries.

http://directory.google.com/Top/Business/Transportation_and_Logistics/Bus/Operators/North_America/

For a list of tour companies with their Internet sites from all over the country.

www.HouseCarers.com

A free service for homeowners. Visit the site for information about postings and how to register for positions throughout the United States.

www.housesitworld.com

Information about house-sitting throughout the world.

www.journeywoman.com

JourneyWoman.com offers resources and articles to adventurous women over 50.

www.mustcruise.com/cruise_info/seniors.html

www.ntaonline.com

To contact the National Tour Association (NTA) for recommendations about a dependable tour company in your area, call 800-682-8886.

www.odysseysunlimited.com

Odysseys Unlimited offers a free catalog about small tour experiences geared toward seniors.

www.poshnosh.com

Senior Travel trips for women who are 50+.

www.ricksteves.com

Rick Steves is famous for his *Europe Through the Back Door* country guides, city guides, and acclaimed video/DVD series. Check his website for all resources.

www.seniorjournal.com/travel

Travel news and information for senior citizens and baby boomers

www.seniorstravelguide.com

Information on top travel destinations in the U.S. and Canada.

www.smarterliving.com/senior

Smarter Living's Senior Travel website offers travel tips, articles about various destinations, and valuable information about deals and discounts specifically for the senior citizen. Sign up for the free *Senior Travel E-Newsletter* to learn about late-booking travel discounts.

www.smartertravel.com/senior-travel

Smarter Travel summarizes the best discounts and specials on airfare, hotels, cruises, tours, and packages.

www.smithsonianjourneys.com

Travel with expert leaders on educational tours.

www.suddenlysenior.com/travelpage.html

Suddenly Senior offers travel tips, bargains, and entertaining stories.

www.thirdage.com/fun

Third Age Travel is a companion matching service and a resource guide for its online visitors. Geared toward seniors, it features travel-related subjects.

www.travmatix.com

Travmatix.com maps out your route, describes conveniences at every roadway exit, including hotels and all their amenities—complimentary breakfast, pools, exercise rooms, wheelchair access, laundry, pet-friendly rooms, data ports, and coffee makers. It also names restaurants in the area and whether they feature play areas, buffets, salad bars, and RV parking.

www.travelocity.com

Sponsored by the AARP, this is a must-visit site before planning a trip.

www.travelwithachallenge.com

*Travel with a Challenge* web magazine is a global travel resource. "Attracting 940,000 readers per year, the 5-year-old publication is updated monthly and speaks directly to the mature/senior traveler. The site offers excellent articles and breaking news about the world. It is a must-visit site before planning your itinerary."

www.tripspot.com

Work with a tour operator who specializes in senior travel.

www.ucanhealth.com

UcanHealth allows disabled travelers can look at equipment that will make travel easier.

www.walkingtheworld.com

Walking the World is adventure travel for people over 50 with walking being the primary mode of transportation. What a great way to experience a country and its natives.

www.wiredseniors.com

Wired Seniors is an excellent website of special interest to seniors. Under *Senior Search*, there is a section on tours featuring senior friendly itineraries.

## Chapter 6
## Pay Back: *The Amazing Rewards and Opportunities of Volunteering*

### Books

Campbell, Katherine H., and Susan J. Ellis. *By the People: A History of Americans as Volunteers*. Philadelphia: Energize Inc., 2005.

Graham, Margaret, and Robert A. Stebbins. *Volunteering as Leisure*. Oxfordshire, UK: CABI Publishing, 2004.

Scheier, Ivan H. *Building Staff/Volunteer Relations*. Philadelphia: Energize Inc., 2003.

### Websites

www.1-800-VOLUNTEER.org; phone: 1-800-volunteer
www.adoptagrandparent.org.
www.eldercarelocator.org; phone: 1-800-677-1116
Faith in Action: www.fiavolunteers.org; phone: 877-324-8411
Global Volunteers: www.globalvolunteers.org; phone: 1-800-487-1074
www.govolunteer.org
www.greenvol.com
www.idealist.org
www.joinseniorservice.org.
Medicare: www.medicare.gov
Meals on Wheels: www.mowaa.org
National Association of Home Care: www.nahc.org; phone: 202-547-7424
National Hospice Organization: www.nhpco.org; phone: 1-800-658-8898

Ombudsman program: www.ombudsman.com; phone: 1-800-252-2412
American Red Cross: www.redcross.org; phone: 1-866-438-4636
Senior Corps: www.seniorcorps.org; phone: 1-800-424-8867
www.serviceleader.org
    ServiceLeader.org is a project of the RGK Center for Philanthropy and Community Service at the Lyndon B. Johnson School of Public Affairs of the University of Texas at Austin, which provides information on all aspects of volunteerism; phone: 404-627-4303.
www.irissoft.com/uwsa
United Way
Visiting Nurses Association: www.vnaa.org; phone: 1-202-384-1420
www.volunteermatch.org
U.S. Government Volunteer Services: www.usafreedomcorp.gov

### Other

National Wildlife Refuge System
4401 N. Fairfax Drive, Room 634
Arlington, VA 22203
Phone: (703) 358-2386; Fax: (703) 358-2517

*Other Federal organizations include:*
The USA Freedom Corps
U.S. Army Corps of Engineers
Department of Veteran Affairs
Cooperative State Research
Corporation for National and Community Service.
Systems Administrator with the Department of the Interior:
    Douglas_J_Blankinship@ios.doi.gov, or by mail at: Douglas J. Blankinship, Volunteer.Gov/Gov Systems Administrator
    United States Department of the Interior
    1849 C Street, N.W. Mail Stop 5258
    Washington, DC 20240

## Chapter 7
## Grandparenting: *The Best of All Possible Worlds*

### Books

Bosak, Susan V. *How to Build the Grandma Connection.* The Legacy Project at www.legacyproject.org.
Gray, William. *Travel with Kids.* Bath, UK: Footprint Handbooks, 2007.
House Hushion. *Have Grandchildren Will Travel.* New York: Pilot Books, 1997.

Lansky, Vicki. *101 Ways to Make Your Child Feel Special, 101 Ways to Tell Your Child "I Love You," 101 Ways to be a Special Dad,* and *101 Ways to be a Special Mom,* visit www.practicalparenting.com, or call 800-255-3379 to order these books.

## Websites

www.aaa.com

www.aarp.org/travel

www.ancestry.com

www.blogger.com

www.blogster.com

www.createblog.com

www.cyberparent.com

www.disneytravel.com

www.elderhostel.org; phone: 1-877-426-8056

Thomson Family Adventures: www.familyadventures.com; phone:
   1-800-262-6255

www.grandparenting.org

www.grandtravel.com; phone: 1-800-247-7651

www.livejournal.com

www.myheritage.com/familytree

www.nationalgeographicexpeditions.com

www.practicalparenting.com

www.rascalsinparadise.com

www.safekids.org

www.smartdraw.com

www.travelwithgrandkids.com

www.savingsbonds.gov; phone: 1-800-4USBond

## Resorts

Almond Village Resorts
Barbados
phone: 1-800-ALMOND
www.almondresorts.com

Amelia Island Plantation Resort
Florida
phone: 888-261-6161
www.aipfl.com

Atlantis
Paradise Island, Bahamas
phone: 888-528-7155
www.atlantis.com

ClubMed
phone: 1-800-CLUBMED
www.clubmed.com

The Franklyn D. Resort and FDR Pebbles
Jamaica
phone: 1-800-654-1FDR
www.fdrholidays.com

## Cruise Lines

Cruises Only
phone: 1-888-278-4737
www.cruiseline.com

Carnival Cruises
phone: 1-888-CARNIVAL
www.carnival.com

Disney Cruise Line
phone: 1-800-951-3532
www.disney.com

Holland America
phone: 1-800-932-4259
www.hollandamerica.com

Norwegian Cruise Line
phone: 1-800-327-7030
www.ncl.com

Princess Cruises
phone: 1-800-774-6237
www.princesscruises.com

Royal Caribbean
phone: 1-800-398-9819
www.royalcaribbean.com

## Gifts for Grandkids

www.babiesonline.com
www.banananana.com
www.bearsinchairs.com/grandkid.html
www.boomergirl.com/stories
www.cafepress.com
www.designergifts.com/kid.html
www.discoverychannelstore.com
www.everythinggrandkids.com
www.giftsforyounow.com/Children_47.aspx
www.grandkidsgiftguide.com
www.grandtimes.com
www.leapfrog.com
www.literaryguild.com
www.suite101.com
www.thriftyfun.com
www.umdagifts.com

## Videos and CDs

*For the Love of World Travel* (ages 0–4)
*The A to Z Symphony* (ages 0–5)
*Baby Road Trip Jungle* (ages 6 months–4 years)
*We Sign Play Time* (ages 10 months–4 years)
*Brainy Baby* series inspires learning (ages 6 months–5 years)
*All By Myself: Taking Care of My Pet* (ages 2–5)
*Nursery Tap, Hip to Toe Volume One* (ages 2–7)
*Imagination Movers Stir it Up* (ages 2–7)
*Cinderella and More Beloved Fairy Tales* (ages 3–9)
*The Man Who Walked Between the Towers and More Inspiring Tales* (ages 5–10)
*We Sign: Interactive DVDs teach American Sign Language* (ASL) (grades Pre–K+). This is particularly important to learn as ASL meets the language requirement on the high school level.
*Families of the World* (ages 5–11)
*StoryWatchers Club – Adventures in Storytelling* (ages 5–12)
*SpaceTrekkers* (ages 6–10)
*Best Ever Sleepover!* (ages 6 –12)

*Look Mom! I Have Good Manners* (ages 6+)
*Learn Magic with Lyn* (ages 7+)
*The Feeling Good Concert* (ages 11 and under)

## Electronic Educational Products

LeapFrog Fly Through Spelling (grades 3–5)
LeapFrog 100 Hoops Basketball Counting Game (ages 3–6+)
Story Reader books read aloud as you turn the pages (ages 3–8)
LeapPad Plus Writing and Microphone Learning System (ages 4–8)
LeapPad Letter Factory Game (Pre-K–Kindergarten)
LeapFrog LEAPSTER Multimedia Learning System (ages 4–10)
LeapFrog Fly Through Math Multiplication and Division (grades 4–6)
LeapFrog Fly Through Spanish Pocket Translator (ages 8+)
LeapFrog Fly Pentop Computer (ages 8+)
GeoSafari Laptop Expansion Cards for (ages 8+)
LeapPad Learning System (ages 8–11)

## Unique Gifts

Mega Bloks (ages 1–8+)
My First 3 Nature Games (ages 3+)
Great Big Sneaky Puzzle (ages 3+)
Big Brother and Big Sister Kits (ages 3–8)
Matchbox Mega Rig Wrecking Rig (ages 4+)
Junior Mentalogy: The Mind-Expanding Game (ages 4+)
3D Labyrinth (ages 4–8)
Binoculars for Kids (ages 5+)
GeoSafari B.S.I. – Bug Scene Investigator (ages 5+)
GeoSafari Talking Microscope (ages 5+)
Baskin-Robbins Double Scoop Ice Cream Shop (ages 5+)
LEGO City Passenger Plane (ages 5–12)
Safari Rush Hour (ages 6+)
Nifty Plates from the Fifty States (ages 6+)
Tri-Words Game (ages 6+)
LEGO Designer Set Buildings (ages 6+)
Children's Talking Dictionary (ages 6–10)
LEGO Creator Revvin' Riders (ages 7–13)
Cogno: The Alien Adventure Game (ages 7+)
Swap (ages 7+)
LEGO Dino Attack: Iron Predator vs. T-Rex (ages 7–14)
LEGO Tower of Toa (ages 7–15)
Rush Hour Traffic Jam Game (ages 8+)
Mandala Mosaic Magnetic Art (ages 8+)

Lewis & Clark Adventure Game (ages 8+)
Santa Fe Flyer Electric Train Set (ages 8+)
NASCAR Winner's Cup Electric Slot Racing Set (ages 8+)
Tons of Trivia Game (ages 8+)
LEGO Factory Skyline (ages 8+)
Toss Up! (ages 8+)
Mars Science Cards (ages 10+)
Hubble Science Cards (ages 10+)
Perfume Science Experiment Kit (ages 10+)
Malarky Game (ages 10+)
Buzzword (ages 10+)
Captio CollegeCase: College Organizer
Captio AppliCase: College Application Organizer

## Books as Gifts

*The Me Book* (ages infants–preschool)
*Eloise Wilkin Stories* (Little Golden Book Treasury) (ages baby–preschool)
*Big Annie: An American Tall Tale* (Pre-K to 2nd Grade)
*How the Turtle Got Its Shell: An African Tale* (Pre-K to 2nd Grade)
*The Many Adventures of Pengey Penguin* (ages 4+)
*How to Be a Baby by Me, The Big Sister* (ages 4–8)
*Your Father Forever* (ages 4–8)
*Ready, Set, Preschool!* (ages 4–8)
*Alphabet Explosion!: Search and Count from Alien to Zebra* (ages 4–8)
*Our Community Garden* (ages 4–8)
*The 39 Apartments of Ludwig van Beethoven* (ages 4–9)
*The Ballad of Blue Eagle* (ages 4–8)
*Dona Flor: A Tall Tale About a Giant Woman with a Great Big Heart*
    (ages 4–8)
*The True Story of Stellina* (ages 5+)
*The Tailor's Gift, A Holiday Tale for Everyone* (ages 5–7)
*Uneversaurus (A unique look at dinosaurs)* (ages 5–8)
*Jackie and the Shadow Snatcher* (ages 5–8)
*Where Did Daddy's Hair Go?* (ages 5–8)
*1-2-3 Draw* (ages 5–9+)
*The American Story: 100 True Tales from American History* (ages 6+)
*Small Beauties: The Journey of Darcy Heart O'Hara* (ages 6+)
*Junie B., First Grader* (ages 6–9)
*Disney Fairies series* (ages 7–10)
*Toys Go Out* (ages 7–11)
*Anatole* (reading level ages 9–12)
*The Random House Dinosaur Travel Guide* (ages 9–12)

*Kidz Can Do: What Every Person Should Know About Personal Safety*
(ages 9+)

## Chapter 8
## Age-Proofing Your Home: *Create a Safe Environment*

**Books**

Bakker, Rosemary. *Elderdesign.* New York: Penguin Books, 1997.

Buettner, Helmust. *Mayo Clinic on Vision and Eye Health: Practical Answers on Glaucoma, Cataracts, Macular Degeneration & Other Conditions.* New York: Mayo Clinic Trade Paper, 2002.

Gardner, Gerald, and Jim Bellows. *80: Our Most Famous 80 Year Olds.* Gallatin, TN: Source Books, Inc., 2007.

Gillick, Muriel R. *The Denial of Aging: Perpetual Youth, Eternal Life and Other Dangerous Fantasies.* Boston: Presidents and Fellow of Harvard College, 2006.

Meyer, Maria, and Paula Derr. *Comfort of Home: A Complete Guide for Caregivers.* Portland, OR: Care Trust Publications, 2007.

Rubin, Lillian. *60 on Up: The Truth About Aging in America.* Boston: Beacon Press, 2007.

Styne, Marlys Marshall. *Reinventing Myself: Memoirs of a Retired Professor.* Conshohocken, PA: Infinity Publishing, 2006.

**Websites**

CAPS (Children of Aging Parents): www.caps4caregivers.org; phone: 1-800-227-7294

Caregiver Survival Resources: www.caregiver911.com

National Association of Professional Geriatric Care Managers: www.caremaager.org

www.carepathways.com

Centers for Medicare and Medicaid Services: www.cms.gov; phone: 1-800-633-4227

Eldercare Locator: www.eldercare.gov; phone: 1-800-677-1116

www.fashionablecanes.com/caneinfo.htm#fit

U.S. Federal Emergency Management Administration (FEMA): www.usfa.fema.gov

www.medicare.gov

The National Council on the Aging: www.ncoa.org

www.senioremporium.com

United Seniors Council: www.unitedseniorshealth.org; phone: 1-800-637-2604

Wishes on Wheels: www.wishesonwheels.com of phone: 1-800-535-3063

## Chapter 9
## Safety on the Road: *To Drive or Not to Drive?*

### Websites

www.aarp.org/drive

AARP Driver Safety Program: www.aarp.org/families/driver_safety; phone: 1-888-227-7669

American Medical Association Guidelines for Older Drivers: www.ama-assn.org/ama/pub/category/8925.html

American Occupational Therapy Association: www.aota.org

Certified Driver Rehabilitation Specialists: www.driver-ed.org

Eye Care America: phone: 1-800-222-3937

Insurance Institute for Highway Safety: www.iihs.org

The Defensive Driving School: www.thedefensivedrivingschool.com

www.thehartford.com/talkwitholderdrivers/having/conversopeners .htm

## Chapter 10
## Avoiding Scams and Fraud: *Refuse to be a Victim*

### Books

Alt, Betty L., and Sandra K. Wells. *Fleecing Grandma and Grandpa: Protecting Against Scams, Cons and Frauds.* Oxford, UK: Praeger Publishers, 2004.

Kirchheimer, Sid. *Scam Proof Your Life: 377 Ways to Protect You and Your Loved Ones from Rip-offs, Bogus Deals and Other Consumer Headaches.* New York: Sterling Publishing, 2006.

Stossel, John. *Give Me A Break: How I Exposed Huckster, Cheats, Scam Artists and Became the Scourge of the Liberal Media.* New York: Harper Collins, 2004.

### Websites

Consumer Product Safety Commission: www.cpsc.gov/cpscpub

Council of Better Business Bureau: www.bbb.org; phone: 703-276-0100

Do Not Call registry: www.DONOTCALL.GOV; phone: 888-382-1222

Eldercare Locator: www.eldercare.gov

Information: www.211.org; phone 211

United Way

www.irissoft.com/uwsa

www.nationalconsumersleague.com

National Consumers League; phone: 1-800-355-9625

www.officialscambusters.blogspot.com

www.scambuster.org

www.snopes.com

## Chapter 11
## Taking Control: *Safety Away From Home*

### Books

Butler, Robert N. *The Longevity Revolution: The Benefits and Challenges of Living a Long Life,* New York: Perseus Publishing, 2008.

Butler, Robert N. *Why Survive Being Old in America.* Baltimore: The John Hopkins University Press, 1975.

Cruikshank, Margaret. *Learning to Be Old: Gender, Culture, and Aging.* Lanham, MD: Rowman & Littlefield Publishers, Inc., 2002.

Gullette, Margaret Morgaroth. *Aged by Culture.* Chicago: University of Chicago Press, 2004.

Nelson, Todd D. *Ageism: Stereotyping and Prejudice Against Older Persons.* Boston: First MIT Press, 2004.

Palmore, Erdman Ballagh. *Ageism: Negative and Positive.* New York: Springer Publishing Company, 1999.

### Websites

Department of Aging and Disability Services: www.aasa.dshs.wa.gov; phone: 800-422-3263

Jitterbug cell phones: www.jitterbug.com; phone: 800-918-8543

Social Security Administration fraud line: www.socialsecurity.gov; phone 800-269-0271

www.usfa.fema.gov

## Chapter 12
## Depression, Fear, and Grief: *Conquering the Challenges of Aging*

### Books

Bylock, Ira. *Dying Well: Defining Wellness Through the End of Life.* New York: Berkley Publishing Group, 2002.

Cornils, Stanley. *Your Healing Journey Through Grief: A Practical Guide to Grief Management.* Bandon, OR: Robert D. Reed Publishers, 2002.

Hickman, Martha W. *Healing after Loss: Daily Meditation for Working Through Grief.* New York: Avon Book, 1994.

James, John W. *The Grief Recovery Handbook: A Step-by-Step Program for Moving Beyond Loss.* New York: Harper Collins, 1998.

Jay, Debra, and Carol Colleran. *Aging and Addiction: Helping Older Adults Overcome Alcohol or Medication Dependence.* Hazelden, MN: Authors, 2002.

Kubler-Ross, Elizabeth. *On Grief and Grieving: Finding the Meaning of Grief Through the Five Stages of Loss.* New York: Simon & Schuster, 2005.

Neeld, Elizabeth H. *Seven Choices: Taking the Steps to a New Life after Losing Someone You Love.* Online: IBS Books, 1997.

Rando, Therese A. *How to Go On Living When Someone You Love Dies.* Lanham, MD: Lexington Books, 1988.

Westberg, Granger, E. *Good Grief.* Minneapolis, MN: Fortress Press, 2005.

**Websites**

American Association of Retired People (AARP): www.aarp.org/life/griefandloss; phone: 888-687-2277

www.caringinfo.org

Alcoholics Anonymous: www.alcoholicsanonymous; phone: 800-593-3330

American Hospice Foundation: www.americanhospice.org

Center to Advance Palliative Care: www.capc.org

Elder Abuse Center: www.elderabusecenter.org

Elder Abuse Prevention: www.elderabuseprevention.com

Elder Care Locator: www.eldercare.org; phone: 800-677-1116

Elder Rage: www.elderrage.com

Hospice Foundation: www.hospicefoundation.org; phone: 800-658-8898

National Hospice and Palliative Care Organization: www.nhpco.org

Share the Care: www.sharethecare.org

www.practicalbioethics.org

*Caring Conversations.* The Center for Practical Bioethics; phone: 800-344-3829 to order the workbook

The National Institutes of Health: www.niaaa.nih.gov; call Focus on Recovery; phone: 800-234-0420.

## Chapter 13
## Gratitude: *Honoring Those We Love*

**Books**

Breathnach, Sarah Ban. *Simple Abundance.* New York: Warner Books, 1995.

Brickey, Michael. *Defy Aging: Develop the Mental and Emotional Vitality to Live Longer.* Columbus, OH: NewResources Press, 2000.

Byron, Katie, and Stephen Mitchell. *Loving, What Is It: Four Questions That Can Change Your Life.* New York: Three Rivers Press, 2002.

Gottman, John M. *Seven Principles for Making a Marriage Work.* New York: PRD Group, 1999.

Gottman, John M. *The Relationship Cure: A Five-step Guide for Building Better Communication.* New York: Three Rivers Press, 1999.

Lowery, Fred. *The Covenant Marriage: Staying Together For Life.* West Monroe, LA: Howard Publishing Company, 2002.

## Websites

www.allmothersdaygifts.com
www.beyondbookmarks.com
www.caregiver.com
www.dynamic-living.com
www.eldercareteam.com
www.elderluxe.com
www.everythingmothersday.com
www.findgift.com
www.firststreetonline.com
www.gifts.com
www.giftsforseniors.com
www.giftideasforseniors.com
www.grannyjoproducts.com
www.overstock.com
www.poetspassion.com
www.rehabilitystores.com
www.senioremporium.com
www.seniorshops.com
www.seniorstore.com
www.silverts.com
www.songsender.com
www.storycorps.net
www.theholidayspot.com/mothersday
www.thingsremembered.com
www.wellhaven.com
www.wiredseniors.com
www.zazzle.com

# Index